HEALTH
Search & Rescue

by
Sarah King Feldman

Health Search & Rescue

By Sarah King Feldman, N.C.

For related titles and support materials, visit our online catalogue at www.foodbeautiful.com

Cover and book design by Renee Lundquist
Back cover photo by Travis Daniels Photography www.travisdphotography.com

Full color interior: ISBN 1453880747
Black and white interior: ISBN 1456494686
First printing, December 2010

CIP data available from the Library of Congress

PRINTED IN THE UNITED STATES OF AMERICA

Health Search & Rescue

by Sarah King Feldman

CONTENTS

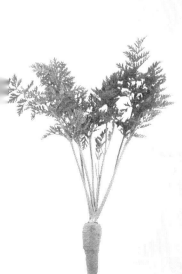

I am deeply grateful for those who have contributed to the book's completion:

The creator of the universe YHVH, my husband Will, my father Michael King,
my book designer Renee Lundquist, and my editors Liz Calhoun and Katherine Szerdy.
Thank you!

Thank you also to all my family, friends and clients for your support and constant encouragement.

Dying to Be Told – My Father's Cancer Battle

The story behind the inception of the writing of this book started during my freshman year at the University of Colorado at Boulder. I was fairly confident that everything in my life would be flawless--no bumps--just a smooth road ahead. Little did I know that one phone call later, my "perfect" life would drastically change. I was in for the worst shock of my life.

Fall semester was coming to a close, and I was anticipating a relaxing winter break with my family, when minutes before my final exam in biology I received a call from my mom. Without delay, she blurted out, "Your dad has been diagnosed with stage three colon cancer, and he is scheduled to have surgery next week." I was speechless. After a few moments of gathering my thoughts, I replied, "But he's never been sick in his life. I don't understand!" At that point all I knew about cancer was that it was a horrific disease that kills thousands every year.

I just couldn't believe that my dad was sick! He had never been sick before, he wasn't over-weight, he ran every day, and he loved God with all his heart. I thought for a moment, then said to my mother, "He couldn't have cancer; it doesn't run on his side of the family!"

The truth was that he had done nothing to prevent cancer. At that point the only education he had received about health was from his doctor and through mainstream media. He was taught that when you get sick, you go to the doctor, he gives you some pills, and in a couple of days you might feel better. This time a pill wouldn't fix the damage.

I became an emotional wreck that week but somehow pulled myself together to finish the semester. All I wanted was to be right beside my dad. All my concentration was on worrying about what might happen to him. My mom called every hour with updates which did nothing more than fuel my fear about what was going to happen. My father was told the only way to attempt recovery was to have a colon resection, involving the removal of a 12-inch section of his colon, followed by aggressive chemotherapy. Out of fear and desperation, he plunged into what almost became his death sentence, with complete faith that the doctors would fix everything.

By the third dose of chemotherapy my dad was on his deathbed. My unbreakable father was broken; he lost over 50 pounds in less than a month. He had gone from being an independent, completely self-motivated father to a frail man needing assistance with basic bodily functions. I saw my father-- a confident, dignified man—become completely demoralized and vulnerable in a matter of days.

It wasn't long before he began to realize that he wasn't dying from the cancer but from the chemotherapy. Fortunately for my father, Western medicine wasn't working! This is ultimately what led him to find a cure through His Creator's healing method.

My dad's first step toward recovery began with a shift of his mindset. He began to believe in the divine power that the Creator had given him; the innate wisdom of the human body to heal itself. Despite his doctors' recommendations, he chose to stop all prescribed medical treatments. He set forth on a journey to reeducate himself on alternative healing practices and hired a naturopathic doctor to assist him in his healing process. He threw himself into research, spending hours every day studying health books, researching online, and learning from nutritional experts.

His second step toward recovery was to complete a seven-day cleanse, nearly identical to the "Total Body Cleanse" in Chapter 3, to purge his body of toxic waste. His third step was to consume a minimum of 48-60 ounces of fresh juices and raw plant-based foods. He transformed an 80% cooked diet into an 80% raw diet. He adopted proper food combining principles, eliminated all animal-based foods, flour, and sugar, used proper supplementation, and drank only purified water. One month after changing his lifestyle his energy had tripled and he looked 15 years younger than before his surgery. That was a "wow" factor for our entire family and my father's oncologist. After five months on the new program my dad requested a colonoscopy. His doctors were stunned at the results, as they were negative. Since 1997 he has been 100% cancer-free.

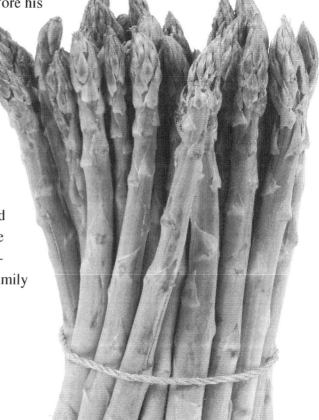

My father's complete health turn-around is the essence of the Food Beautiful lifestyle presented in this book. Take some time to observe how the standard American lifestyle and diet has encouraged disease and sickness to manifest in your family and friends around you. This book can dramatically change the way you and your loved ones overcome or prevent disease.

A goal without a plan is just a wish! This book is a plan that can be easily followed.

During my father's recovery, I saw firsthand how raw plant-based foods and a sound mind can free the human body from disease. My father's victory over cancer ignited a passion in me for the truth and results of a holistic lifestyle. I was determined to learn the pathways in which the body becomes sick and how to restore healthy pathways without medicine. I spent my time daily investigating medical journals, health articles and books, diet plans, homeopathic books, and integrative nutrition to start piecing everything together. This was just the beginning of my journey into discovering true health and where it can be found. My father's crisis and recovery proves to science that no matter what doctors say about your state of health, you ultimately have the choice and power to take the necessary action to heal yourself.

This book is the culmination of the research I've done and knowledge I've acquired in the field of holistic health and nutrition. As you read through the Food Beautiful principles, understand that these principles are nearly identical to "the plan" my father used to cure himself of cancer. I pray that this information will give you freedom of choice and action and equip you to share these truths with your friends and family, so others won't have to go through what my father went through.

May the words of this book bring forth action, and ultimately, complete health to every cell in your body!

Principle 1

Overcome your toxic mindset and behaviors

The foundations of a sound diet begin with a healthy mind! What sets you apart from someone who is fit, youthful, vibrant, and healthy? The difference is that their mind believes they deserve and can achieve the goal they desire. Your mind is a powerful force that translates thoughts into their physical counterparts. Your inner thoughts and beliefs, coupled with their correlating actions, bring you either abundance or limitation. So if you believe yourself to be fat, ugly, poor, sick, and worthless, you will be just that. Begin today to let go of past failures. Your mind is powerful--harness its ability to believe and receive your desired outcome.

Begin by changing your thoughts and beliefs from what you don't want to what you do want. And be specific! For example: "I will overcome my sickness in three months' time by drinking 48 ounces or more of Food Beautiful juices, and by seeking to forgive myself and my mother." Whatever your goal may be, write it down and say it daily. It doesn't matter if you don't know the exact way to achieve your goal. That will come. Focus on believing that your goal will be accomplished. Activate the power of your mind to manifest your desire by visualizing, emotionalizing, believing, and acting upon those goals. Use the intention rock

> Keep your thoughts positive because your thoughts become your words. Keep your words positive because your words become your behaviors. Keep your behaviors positive because your behaviors become your habits. Keep your habits positive because your habits become your values. Keep your values positive because your values become your destiny.
>
> - Mahatma Gandhi

mentioned earlier or find a deeper reason why you must change. When you start to think negative thoughts, stop yourself. Say out loud, "Stop," and then say what you want to do. You may not do it perfectly, but over the course of 21 days you will have solidified the action of good habits. Your life is the exact mirror of your inner self-talk. It may seem like a chore at first to monitor your mind, but soon you will retrain your subconscious to believe you can achieve anything.

Aligning your thoughts with your desires allows your life to naturally attract your goal. Martin Luther said, "Take the first step in faith; you don't have to see the whole staircase, just take the first step."

PRINCIPLE 1 ACTION STEP:

Start making a list of goals: two to three things you want to receive and achieve this month, in six months, and in one year. Write these goals down and post them in a place where you can see them every day. Be specific and clear about your goals. Then set aside time every night when you have no distractions, and allow your mind to nurture and manifest your desires. Spend this time visualizing and emotionalizing these goals and desires. These sentences should be positive assertions beginning with words like, "I am…", "I do…", or "I overcome…" Soon your mind will start to believe, and you will start becoming what you have always wanted to become. Then allow God to continue empowering your mind, building up in you the belief in the promise of his blessings for you. Memorize your goals so that if someone woke you up in the middle of the night asking you, "What do you want most in life?" you could answer without a moment's hesitation.

Principle 2

Drink & Shower with Purified Water–Look and Feel Younger!

Hydrating with tap water or unfiltered waters can cause your body to become a breeding tank for devastating sicknesses. The simple act of properly hydrating the body is extremely difficult due to the myriad of harmful chemicals and bacteria in our water today. However, using properly structured filtered water or fresh spring water can bring healing and life to every cell in your body.

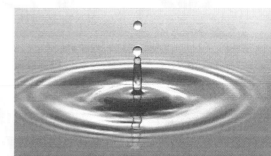

What exactly is in our water that makes it so unsafe? It is easy to find harmful amounts of chlorination byproducts, fluoride, hormones, pharmaceutical drugs (including narcotics, birth control, antibiotics, antidepressants, and the like), cancer-causing nitrates, fungus, mold, feces, viruses, parasites, pesticides, heavy metals, radioactive compounds, and petrochemicals in nearly all local municipal water supplies. If you get your water from a private well, all contaminants except for the chlorination byproducts may be present. The toxins and free radicals in these waters are made significantly more toxic to humans by the addition of chlorine, a compound mandated by local public health departments. The Environmental Protection Agency now reports that individuals who drink and bathe in chlorinated surface waters (i.e., water from lakes, rivers and shallow wells) have a 50% greater likelihood of getting cancer in their lifetime. [1][2][3]

Your body is comprised of over 75% water, your brain 83% water and your blood 84% water. Water is an essential element in all physiological functions of the body—you can't live without it! In fact, if your body drops below 1% of normal hydration it will begin to lose ability to function.

Drinking impure water is one thing. But what about showering in it? It may surprise you to learn that your body can absorb up to 600% more contaminants in a ten-minute shower than in all the tap water consumed in a day. Chlorine gas was banned from warfare long ago, but each bath or shower you take contains the same substance.

> **Many health institutes, doctors, sports and fitness centers, and clinics around the world are now recommending using high quality purification systems.**

In addition to consuming and showering in impure water, the majority of people drink junk liquids that are caffeinated, carbonated, and alcoholic, causing the body to manifest life-threatening illnesses in bizarre ways. Improper hydration translates into diseases like high blood pressure, high cholesterol, thyroid disorders, liver disease, constipation, autoimmune diseases, fibromyalgia pain, sleep disorders, joint aches, fatigue, hypertension, edema, acne, lupus, migraines, sinusitis, obesity, headaches, allergies, depression, anxiety, Type 2 diabetes, Parkinson's disease, Alzheimer's, lymphoma, angina, heartburn, back pain, colitis, cancer and many more. And, to make matters worse, instead of hydrating with healing water, people often take drugs for these problems that further dehydrate their body and exacerbate their illnesses.

Many health institutes, doctors, sports and fitness centers, and clinics around the world are now recommending using high quality purification systems. Some systems have been shown to remove 99.9999% of contaminants with their multiple layers of crystals, rare stones, and nanocarbons that purify, structure, and enhance the water.

Properly purified water also provides essential trace minerals that naturally occur in spring water to increase your energetic and biological functions. Water treated with filtration has a natural resistance to the growth of harmful bacteria and fungi, increasing the rate of hydration of the skin and tissues, thus accelerating the rate of nutrient absorption into the bloodstream. Users have reported a noticeable increase of energy in all areas of health including improved digestion, elimination, mental clarity, and weight loss. In Japan, many doctors routinely prescribe a spring-like filtration system to their patients to aid the body in fighting specific chronic conditions.

PRINCIPLE 2 ACTION STEP:

Start consuming and showering with purified water that hydrates, protects, nourishes, and heals your body from illness. Drink a minimum of 64 ounces of purified water a day. Shed weight, detoxify, and increase mental function by 40% by drinking 20 ounces of water 20 minutes before meals. Remove carbonated, alcoholic, caffeinated, and sugar-laden beverages from your diet or reduce their consumption to 5% of weekly liquid intake.

"We must pay respect to water, and feel love and gratitude, and receive its vibrations with a positive attitude. Then water changes, you change, and I change. Because both you and I are water."
- *Masaru Emoto*, Author of the New York Times bestseller The Hidden Messages in Water

1 Carlo, George L. "Cancer Incidence and Trihalomethane Concentrations in the Public Drinking Water System." American Journal of Public Health, Vol. 74, No. 5, 479-484, 1984.

2 "Organic Chemical Contaminants in Drinking Water and Cancer." American Journal of Epidemiology, Vol. 110, 420, 1979.

3 Anderson, Ian. "Showers Pose a Risk to Health." New Scientist, September 18, 1986.

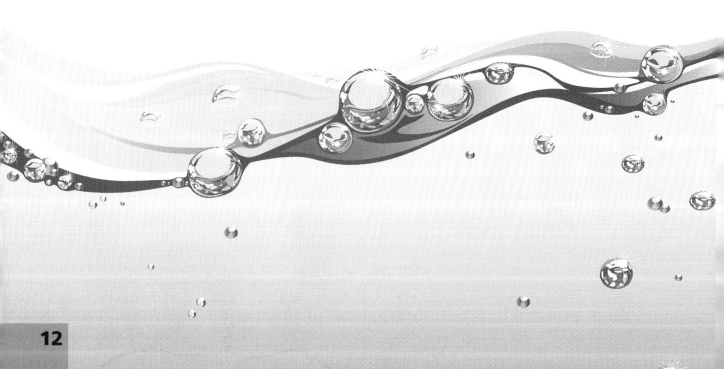

Principle 3

Cleanse the Body–Flush Away Toxins

Since early Biblical times, people have been fasting and cleansing for many reasons including health, political ends, and spiritual enlightenment. However, in our day and age, the average person has no idea about the health benefits fasting and cleansing can provide. Before we can create healthy bodies and minds by eliminating highly toxic foods, it is best to allow the body to clear itself through a process of cleansing. This will raise the vibration of each cell, changing them from magnets for disease to strong guardians of health. The person with a toxin-free body and a sound mind is the person unaffected by epidemics.

Cleansing is an excellent way to rid the body of compacted fecal matter, pesticides, chemicals, parasites, artificial flavors and colors, preservatives, rancid oils and pollutants, viruses, fungi, and unhealthy foods that are stored in various organs, cells, and fat tissue. Symptoms of toxic overload include digestive problems, joint pain, headaches, low energy, allergic reactions, asthma, allergies, anxiety, depression, mental confusion and a host of diseases. Cleansing is an opportunity for new beginnings; it will allow your body to recuperate, renew, and regroup lost energy and health. Cleansing allows the organs to rest from digesting and work on attacking the illness or disease in the body. For optimal health, a cleanse is recommended once in the spring and once in the fall.

> Cleansing is an opportunity for new beginnings; it will allow your body to recuperate, renew, and regroup lost energy and health

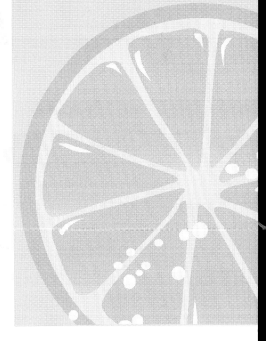

PRINCIPLE 3 ACTION STEP:

If you want to let go of the symptoms or issues listed above, make it your goal to do one of the cleanses in Chapter 3 within the next 21 days. For aggressive cleansing choose the Intensely Clean Total Body Cleanse outlined in Chapter 3. Please use caution if you are attempting a cleanse for the first time, or if you currently have severe symptoms or known toxicity. Consult a healthcare provider before starting any program. When you detoxify and cleanse you will experience greater health, vitality, energy, happiness, clarity, and purpose in life. By cleansing you will naturally progress to eating a clean and healthy diet.

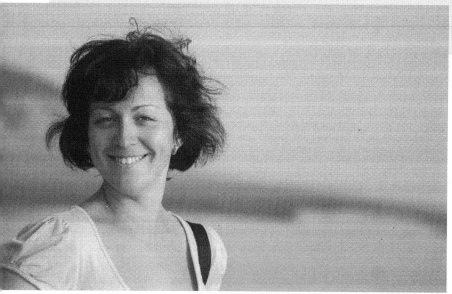

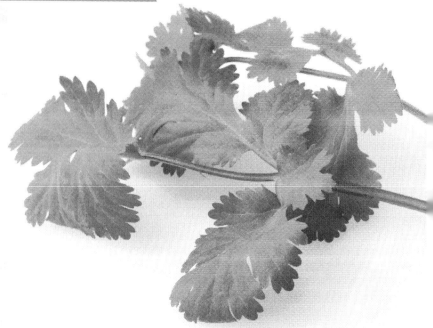

Principle 4

Consume Healing Foods--
Avoid Deceptive Foods

You were created divinely and the earth abounds with foods created to nourish the life of your body. Man-made, processed food is inferior for you! Eating organic, whole foods--foods that are the closest to their original state--will heal and rejuvenate your body. The more raw foods and juices you eat, the more beautiful and healthy you will become.

The first foods into your mouth should be those highest in nutrient density, lowest in acidity, and highest in insoluble and soluble fiber. Meals don't have to be gourmet or complex, though they should be organic, mostly raw and very tasty. For example, when my husband is preparing breakfast, he likes the process quick. So he will make one of my Food Beautiful vegetable juices, healing smoothie meals, or the coconut chia milk found in Chapter 7.

Our philosophy is that every meal should incorporate 80% raw foods--organic fruits, vegetables, sprouts, and nuts or seeds before any other food. Foods that are nutrient-dense control your appetite, blood sugar, and cravings.

It's simple! Following the Food Beautiful Principles will become a habit and a healthy addiction, not a yo-yo diet. You don't need to count calories, just focus on consuming nutrient-dense foods before any other food.

> God said, "See, I have given you every green herb that yields seed which is on the face of all the earth, and every tree whose fruit yields seed; to you it shall be for food."

Listed in order are the foods highest in nutrients per calorie:

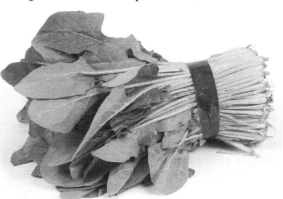

1. Raw Leafy Greens
2. Solid Green Vegetables
3. Non-green Vegetables
4. Beans and Legumes
5. Fresh Fruit
6. Grains
7. Nuts & Seeds

The more green foods and green juices you eat, the healthier and less diseased you will become. Your cells will become less inflamed and acidic. And wonderful side effects include younger looking skin, weight loss, and possibly disease elimination. You will require less food to be satisfied and will feel full much earlier in your meal (as long as you add the green leafy vegetables first). There is a favorable mix of all known essential nutrients found in a balanced whole-food plant-based diet.

Although this principle focuses on what foods are best for you, it is still important to have an understanding of what foods are low in nutrients compared to the top seven, nutrient-dense foods. Low-nutrient foods have an abundance of carbohydrate, fat, and protein calories and are deficient in vitamins, minerals, phytonutrients, essential fatty acids, and amino acids. High calorie foods alone will not satisfy your body's hunger even though they might fill you up. Any weight problem is a result of malnourishment and vitamin deficiency from low nutrient foods. Low-nutrient foods will make you want more food and contribute to poor health, disease, obesity, and fatigue. Some examples of low-nutrient foods are: canned foods, bagels, chips, candy, soda, white rice, white flour, sugar, ice cream, dairy, red meat, chicken, turkey, fried foods, breads, and pastries. Fortunately there are healthier alternatives to low-nutrient foods, which may still be eaten minimally, and only after nutrient-dense foods. Learn more about this in **Chapter 4, Appendix 2: Food Replacements**, and **Appendix 3: First Aid Food Kit--Foods that "Kill the Craving"**.

PRINCIPLE 4 ACTION STEP:

The first foods into your mouth should be those highest in nutrient density. Although this may sound lofty, it is attainable to consume 48 ounces of fresh vegetable juices, and 4 cups of raw leafy greens and orange colored vegetables a day. Eat organic food as much as possible. Omit eating the "fake" and unhealthy foods listed in **Chapter 4**, **Appendix 1**, and **Appendix 2**. Practice adding one new whole-plant based food to your diet each week, while simultaneously removing one toxic food. In the first three weeks of transition, limit your daily allowance of low-nutrient foods to less than 150 calories a day or 1,500 per week. In week 4, limit your intake of low-nutrient foods to three days of 150 calories, and by week five or six choose one day a week where you have one low-nutrient dense food that does not exceed more than 1/3 of your daily calories.

Divide a piece of paper in half. Label the left column "Low-Nutrient Foods" and the right column "Nutrient-Dense Foods." On the left, write a list of the low-nutrient foods you eat for breakfast, lunch, snack, and dinner. On the right, list the nutrient-dense foods with which you will replace the items in the first column. Take your goals list, your food replacement list, and five motivating quotes or goals from this book and tape them to your bathroom mirror, refrigerator, car stereo, computer, cupboard, closet door, and desk at work. Summarize your goals into a short sentence and write it on a keepsake or small colorful rock as a reminder. Then read it every chance you get! Or try to spend 15 minutes each night visualizing yourself doing these things. It is your action that produces the result, and no one else will do it for you.

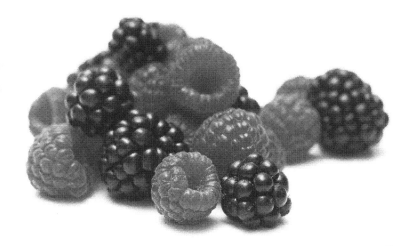

Principle 5

Practice Food Combining and Heal Thyself

Proper food combining is not a new fad or a passing craze. Its earliest roots can be found in ancient Greece and has been practiced in the U.S. by practitioners of Natural Hygiene, a healthcare philosophy practiced for over 150 years. Natural Hygienists believe there are three cycles through which the body operates during a 24-hour period. If these cycles are ignored, confusion is created in the body's systems and a breakdown in function can result.

Since digestion requires so much energy to accomplish, it is logical that we should want it to occur as efficiently as possible. This is where proper food combining is extremely beneficial. If foods are improperly combined, digestion can take up to eight hours to complete, whereas when properly combined, it only takes about three hours.

RULES FOR PROPER FOOD COMBINING

Protein and vegetables combine perfectly. Do not mix starches with proteins.

Starches and vegetables combine perfectly. Do not mix starches with proteins.

Fruits should be eaten alone, in the morning before other foods.

Do not combine fats with proteins. It is okay to combine fat with starches.

Proper food combining saves us a lot of energy for the things we need to do every day like working, playing, detoxifying, and healing. This style of eating prevents fermentation, gas, and bloating in the gut while assisting the healthy metabolism that produces more energy, mental acuteness, and emotional stability so individuals can handle stress more appropriately.

You will learn more in **Chapter 5**!

There are some natural exceptions to the food combining rules. When the rules are applied to your eating style, you will lose weight, start overcoming disease, and look and feel much younger.

PRINCIPLE 5 ACTION STEP:

Make several copies of the **Food Combining Chart** in **Chapter 5** and use it as a guide whenever you are planning meals or eating out—post it in your kitchen and keep a copy in your car, purse, or wallet.

For the first 21 days, choose to either commit three days a week or one meal a day for proper food combining. For the second set of 21 days, commit to five days of proper food combining or two meals each day. By the third set of 21 days, commit to proper food combining six days out of the week. In **Chapter 7** the recipes have a symbol indicating how well that recipe meets the food combining criteria to help you meet your goals.

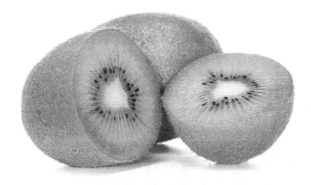

Principle 6

Exercise and Breathe with Intention

Your body is designed to move and work at various intensity levels to produce abundant health, strength, joy, and success in life. We all know we need to exercise, but some of us still ignore this important requirement. If you want an abundant life, you must give energy to get it! When you allow complacency into your life it opens the door to frustration, self-hatred, self-doubt, fear, stress, depression, anger, disease and sickness.

But the good news is you can choose to turn your complacency into action and commitment. Physical action promotes self-love, self-belief, faith, joy, strength, passion, success, and abundance. When you choose to make your health a priority, you begin reaping the benefits of a positive mindset. The more you feel good, the more action you take; it's a self-perpetuating cycle! At any moment you can start a new life with a shift in your thoughts and actions. You can choose to either move forward or sit back and watch your life pass you by. Don't let your past choices or failures keep you from your best future.

Your body was created to adapt to the environment and the stress under which it is placed. Exercise causes you to become stronger, leaner, and healthier. But to avoid injury and to maximize these benefits, this happens in stages. Each time you reach a level to which your body adapts, you must increase the intensity and duration of your exercise, pushing through this uncomfortable stage until you reach your desired health, beauty, and weight. At this point you can maintain your workout schedule.

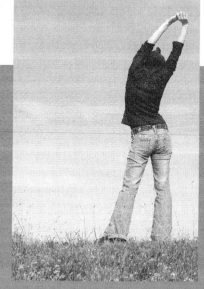

At any moment you can start a new life with a shift in your thoughts and actions. You can choose to either move forward or sit back and watch your life pass you by. Don't let your past choices or failures keep you from your best future.

The key to exercising is to make sure you are doing it effectively, keeping in mind these important variables:

Length of time
Frequency (times you workout per week)
Intensity (workload)
Breathing
Rest

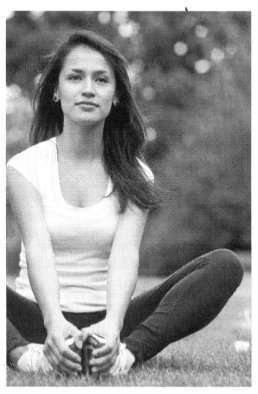

To more accurately measure your fitness level and intensity zone for workouts, you will need to know the following: Maximum Heart Rate, Fat-burning Zone, and Performance Enhancement Rate. You will learn more about these and how to use them in **Chapter 6**.

Over the next six weeks, gradually increase workout time, frequency, and intensity. Then during the seventh week, cut your workout time, frequency, and intensity in half. Then start the cycle all over again. Keep cycling the building periods every six weeks with the seventh week at half the time, frequency, and intensity. There are different types of workouts for various levels of fitness—refer to **Chapter 6** for more details.

PRINCIPLE 6 ACTION STEP:

When you exercise, the energy you invest will result in a stronger, leaner, and healthier you. The key to exercising is to make sure you are doing it effectively, with the proper length of time, frequency, and intensity for your fitness level. Depending on your level of fitness, try to begin the first 21 days by increasing your workout time by 10 minutes a day for three days a week and do the reverse breathing exercises outlined in **Chapter 6** 2-3 times a day for five minutes.

The next 21 days increase your workout by another 10 minutes a day for three days a week. Keep increasing your work load until you hit your goal. Make your goal attainable within 2-3 months. You can achieve your goals using some of the formulas provided in **Chapter 6**.

Principle 7

Eat Delicious Food Beautiful Recipes and Juices

This principle is rather simple—discover how delicious and fun healthy cooking can be while making recipes from this book. Schedule a date cooking night with your spouse or friends and make a dish or two. You can make a dish and take it to a holiday party or weekend party. This way you spread the fun and health that these recipes bring.

There are so many to choose from; just decide where to start and what fits your palate. If you don't like how a recipe turns out or learn a new trick in the process feel free to share that with me at www.foodbeautiful.com.

There are disease-specific lifestyle plans available for purchase at **www.foodbeautiful.com**

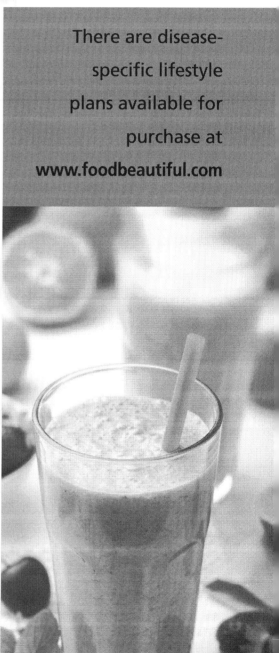

PRINCIPLE 7 ACTION STEP:

Start by planning two days a week to make juices and a recipe from this book. Then make those same juices and that same meal again the next week, so you gain confidence making those recipes. Repeat the process and keep trying new recipes! What I suggest to clients to help them transition into eating healthy, unless dealing with a life-threatening or debilitating disease, is to do as much as possible. For the average health seeker I have them re-place their normal breakfast with a Food Beautiful meal for the first two to three weeks, then replace their lunch or dinner, and by the third set of two to three weeks I have them on an all-Food Beautiful eating style with the allowance of one personal choice day per week. This allows time to adjust and the empowerment to stick with the program.

In the beginning of my father's journey it took him two months to have a solid routine down. Be gracious to yourself. But you must take that first step--and do it now.

True health begins through the application of these seven principles. The chapters in this book are nearly identical to the method in which my father found his healing. His victory over cancer shows that one's health is not found in a pill or at a hospital, but is received when one takes responsibility for his own actions and applies these fundamental principles of life.

For those dealing with a serious illness, you will want to apply all the principles immediately. For those who are just beginning the journey into abundant health you can incorporate one chapter at a time, or multiple sections depending on your level of ability and comfort. Pick up a calendar and write down your monthly goals for each principle/ chapter in this book. Then you will have a written timeline to follow so you can measure your amount of success. Enjoy the learning process provided in this book, and watch as a full measure of success springs up into your life!

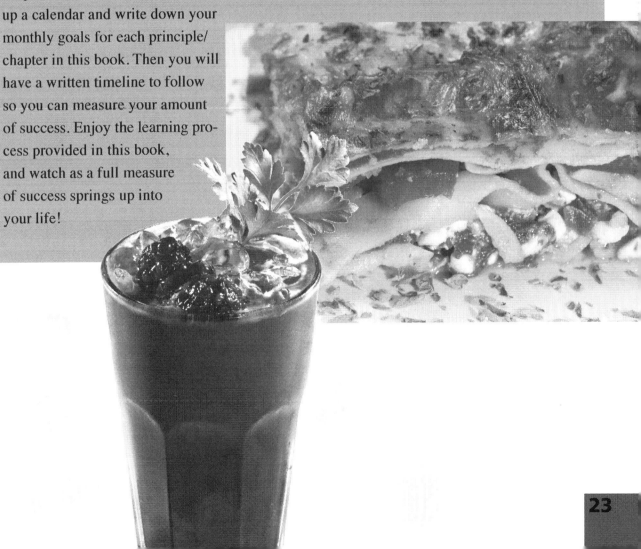

Overcome your toxic mindset and behaviors

You have to get yourself out of the way before you can heal yourself. If you desire to gain true freedom from self-imposed limitations, you have to first recognize that you are not the negative tape playing inside of your head—you are not your disease, addiction or habit. With a shift of inner self-talk and outward actions you can become the person you want to be, free of limitations. The best way to eliminate a toxic mindset is to break the cycle of negative thinking, behavior, and self-limiting actions. This chapter will give you a step by step approach to break the bonds of fear, doubt, self-hatred and disease that have stopped you from reaching your life purpose—mentally, physically and spiritually.

Your mindset is the mental pathway in which you filter, process, and react to your environment (people, places, and things). It originates from, but is not limited to, your life experiences, self-image and relationships. A toxic mindset occurs when a reaction to a common situation in life becomes disruptive for you and the health and safety of others. You have the ability to make choices; not always are you the victim of circumstance. If this were not true, then people would have no hope or ability for good things to happen in their lives.

Family and friends sometimes contribute to a toxic mindset by saturating your mind with unhealthy thoughts, feelings, and actions that suppress your ability to attain success, joy, and health. Surrounding yourself with these sources can poison you with ill feelings like anger, unforgiveness, bitterness, sadness, and jealousy. Limit your time spent with toxic people, avoid agreeing with or affirming antagonizing conversations with them, and learn to find the best characteristics in them. If you cannot change your environment, then find a new one that encourages healthy growth. We all have the ability to choose—you do not have to be the victim! Many times people allow distractions into their lives, enabling the toxic habits that bind them to old behaviors.

It is possible to have a toxic mindset in one area of your life and not in another. You can recognize the toxicity when any type of stressor triggers a negative, unhealthy reaction. Do you see a pattern of behavior that erupts when you are placed in a stressful situation? This chapter sets forth the four steps to change that will guide you to restoring healthy habits, resulting in a healthy mindset.

BEGINNING EXERCISE: MINDSET STONE

Spend some time this week looking for an eye-catching rock or stone, something that grabs your attention and that is small enough to carry in your pocket or wallet. I like to call this the "mindset stone." Later in this chapter you will write down what behavior or mindset you want to have and place that intention onto the "mindset stone". This will serve as a constant reminder of the new change you want manifested. This can help prevent you from backsliding into old habits, while moving you forward toward positive change.

Step 1: Identify Your Self-Limiting Behavior

Once we associate an experience with a feeling, our mind continues to look for evidence that confirms our perception of reality. Just as laws of physics prevent the universe from disintegrating into chaos, so do certain spiritual laws contribute to the quality of our thinking. As we get older, we begin to discover that the old adage is true— experience is the best teacher. If we are willing to look at each experience, encounter, decision, or problem that life presents as an opportunity to learn, that lesson can be used to nurture positive change in ourselves.

To move forward in life you must face the personal fears that control you. Think of it this way: fears can't control, they simply dominate if we let them. Writing down courageous action steps will allow you to choose your mindset instead of reacting. Courage is doing what is required of you even if you fear doing it.

Fear does not have a life of its own, but is "false evidence appearing real," resulting from one's perceptions and only experienced in the mind of the "beholder."

The fear of facing reality can distort your mind's ability to overcome prolems. You may think that a distorted reality will set you free, but this state of denial is intermixing facts with illusions; it is a protective mechanism that allows you to only temporarily avoid the pain. The fact is, avoiding a problem actually prolongs the pain. A seed when planted into the ground has to struggle in order to grow; it must push aside all things that prevent it from blossoming. Otherwise it will die. If you are not blossoming in health, happiness, and success then you may want to start pushing and moving aside the obstacles hindering you. If someone made you mad, tell them. If you are bitter towards a family member, forgive them. If you are sick, eat foods that will bring life to your cells. These actions will allow you to wring out the potential toxins that can form as a result of anger, bitterness, sadness, and the like.

For most of her life, my beautiful sister Alyssa has waged her own personal war against the eating disorder anorexia. At the age of four, she was sexually molested by a neighbor, which robbed her of the innocence and joy of childhood. This evil act left her feeling helpless and vulnerable, which in turn affected her whole mindset.

Limit the environments and stressors you know are unhealthy and this will greatly reduce your risk of having a toxic mindset.

Those suffering from eating disorders subconsciously feel a lack of control over their lives, over their environment, even over their own bodies. Throughout her adolescent years, Alyssa became more serious and withdrawn, eventually requiring in-patient treatment. As she got older, her negative outlook became so ingrained, like a computer stuck in a loop, that it sent her body downward into a spiral of despair. Her mindset enslaved her to destructive lifestyle patterns and behaviors that led her to think that weighing 65 pounds as an adult is normal.

On December 23, 2009, Alyssa checked herself into the Eating Recovery Clinic in Denver. Daily she confronted and processed actions associated to self-mutilating patterns. In part of her therapy she was presented with the decision to forgive the perpetrator for all the pain he caused. For three months a team of counselors and doctors used techniques to create new mental pathways and behaviors to heal her toxic mindset. Although the road to recovery in this serious case has seemed like a long one, Alyssa is now in the process of realizing her worth, discovering that her reality is not what was in her head. The progress we have witnessed is miraculous; a once quiet, withdrawn, frail "little girl" is discovering a life beyond her body. This is life changing—for our entire family! Alyssa is allowing herself the freedom to let go of her toxic behaviors. Not only has she gained healthy weight, she is glowing with purpose and life, maturing into her newfound beauty.

During the process of change, there will be times when you will want to recoil and go back to the way you felt or viewed yourself in the past. Recognize that this is normal, as you discover new pathways that lead to a healthy mindset. Limit the environments and stressors you know are unhealthy and this will greatly reduce your risk of having a toxic mindset.

When a stressor begins to trigger old behaviors, pause your thoughts, look at and touch your "mindset stone", and say that intention out loud. At that very moment you have the choice to choose the new nature over the old. Use your God-given ability to act courageously in spite of fear.

Just like in a game of football there is an offense and a defense. The defense is designed to keep the opposing team from scoring; whereas, the offense is designed to score the touchdown. So let me ask you--who wins the game? The offense or the defense? Whether you are dealing with an addiction, a weight issue, or a serious health condition, your focus must be on the desired outcome (the "touchdown"), not the problem or condition.

According to Webster's dictionary, "reality" is the quality or state of being real; like an event, entity, or state of affair. The state of denial is a refusal to admit the truth or reality.

EXERCISE 1: COLORFUL LITTLE JOURNAL

Pick up a colorful, attractive journal, something you want to write in, and jot down three qualities you like most about yourself, leaving a few blank lines underneath each one. Next, below each word or phrase, write about a time when you exemplified this trait—perhaps during a difficult or painful trial that you worked through. Then, without revealing your list, ask someone close to you to do the same exercise, writing down three traits which they believe best describe you. Compare the two lists and write about how you may unrealistically view yourself. After this, write about what you feel you were put on this earth to do--what makes you unique, set apart from others. Do you see what you want to become? These exercises will act as a buffer between you and the problem(s) or toxins that trigger your toxic mindset.

The human understanding is like a false mirror, which, receiving rays irregularly, distorts and discolors the nature of things by mingling its own nature with it. - *Francis Bacon*

Step 2: Forgive Yourself And Others

Perhaps the individual you most need to forgive is yourself. At the same time there may be some long overdue words of forgiveness for you to give a family member, friend or coworker that you may have hurt or vice versa. In that case, try looking at the situation as though you were an outsider. By taking on the perspective of someone outside the situation, removing yourself from the drama, you may become more merciful toward yourself. The act of forgiveness must involve not only the shift of spiritual perception or attitude, but also a making amends, often taking the form of some kind of outward action. Write a letter, make a phone call, send an email--the words need to be spoken and heard. First take the time to think through what needs to be said so that you avoid further damage. Prayer for spiritual guidance is imperative before taking any action. Obedience to that spiritual guidance is the key to inner healing and fullness of joy. After performing the action of forgiveness of ourselves and others, the behavior of forgiveness needs to be continued. Words mean very little if your following actions indicate the opposite.

Experiencing forgiveness, practicing new behaviors, and becoming free of a toxic mindset all contribute to the retraining of our perception of reality, and we start to learn patterns of love and acceptance. When we start framing our self-talk with positive messages we find the love and comfort similar to what we sought from our parents when we were young. Think back to when you had a childhood illness and you needed the love and comfort of a parent or loved one. The gentle touch of your mother laying a cool washcloth on your forehead, a soft prayer spoken, or the comfort of a warm bowl of soup gave you the reassurance that you would soon be well. Use good times and feelings to remind you of what you are becoming. More than mere positive thinking, this form of self-improvement will put you in the frame of mind to forgive yourself and others. You are an overcomer; the pure desires of your heart will be fulfilled!

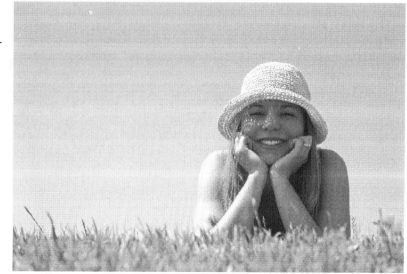

EXERCISE 2: FORGIVENESS

Take your journal out and start writing down the wrongs that you have done to others and the wrongs that have been done to you. If you are feeling resistance towards this exercise, you might want to explore why. Write about your hesitation. You may be amazed at what comes up. When a hurtful memory arises in your mind, pay attention to it, explore the emotions, write down who was involved and how this incident made you feel. After you have completed this exercise, pay attention to how you are feeling both physically and emotionally. You may need to revisit an experience with a relative or classmate who has caused you great pain, leaving you feeling angry, insecure, or rejected. One of the healthiest and most effective ways to move beyond the past and overcome the hurt is to write down your hurts and verbally forgive. Writing about the circumstances surrounding a hurtful situation uncovers what specifically needs to be bathed in prayer and gently turned over to our Creator's loving hands. Sometimes, we have to ask God in prayer for the desire for the desire (no, that is not a typo) to forgive the individual. After journaling, read the entry aloud to yourself, then to God, and finally to a safe and trusted friend.

Step 3: Dump Toxic Habits

Sometimes a toxic mindset is the result not of a wrong committed against you and the resulting bitterness and unforgiveness, but of a lifestyle rooted in aimlessness, lack of focus, or busyness (trying to do too much). If you know in your heart that you were born for more and realize you've been holding yourself back with aimless actions, busyness, and lack of focus, stop it now! Busyness and distractions are the enemies keeping you from a life of power! This type of lifestyle keeps you from experiencing ownership over a project completed or well done. Trying to do too much at one time is called multi-tasking. Research has shown that multi-tasking does not work! Instead, it actually increases the chance of making mistakes and slows you down. David E. Meyer, a cognitive scientist and director of the Brain, Cognition and Action Laboratory at the University of Michigan said, "Multitasking is going to slow you down, increasing the chances of mistakes." Furthermore, "disruptions and interruptions are a bad deal from the standpoint of our ability to process information" (New York Times article "Slow Down Brave Multi-tasker," March 27, 2007.)

EXERCISE 4: PRIORITIZE YOUR LIFE

Begin your day by writing down what needs to be done. Then prioritize your tasks in order of importance, i.e. what tasks needs to be done first, and stay with each task until it is completed. Your success rate for completion of projects will dramatically increase when you write the list down the night before; your subconscious will kick in and begin to create the pathways to reach your goals. Everyone's process for task completion is different, but the outcome is the same--tasks successfully completed.

Step 4: Retrain Your Mind

Reprogramming our neurological pathways through spoken prayer and meditation affirms our new beliefs. Even when we feel weak, we always have the choice to act courageously in spite of how we feel. Feelings are temporal, a false measure of reality. When we approach a stop sign, we don't put the car in park, jump out of the car, grab the stop sign, and carry it with us—instead, we obey the traffic law by stopping, and then move on, leaving the stop sign behind. When we are suffering from illness, depression, or addiction, we tend to take the stop sign--our self-imposed label--with us instead of leaving it where it belongs.

In his book Man's Search for Meaning, psychiatrist and author Viktor Frankl relates his amazing story of survival of four years in Nazi death camps during the Holocaust. Despite the tragic loss of his parents, his brother, and his pregnant wife, Frankl relates how he came to learn that suffering cannot be avoided, yet we always have the ability within our means to choose our response, to learn how to cope, to discover meaning in the midst of trials, and to finally to move forward with a renewed sense of purpose. Viktor Frankl could have given in to despair and depression, but instead he came to realize that the only true freedom resided in his mind. And we have the freedom to choose our attitude--to change our mindset, and to daily feed that change

In a recent study, it took Microsoft workers, on average, 15 minutes to return to serious mental tasks after receiving and responding to incoming e-mail or instant messages. Trying to do too much actually eats up your time. Start by staying focused with what you are doing, avoid procrastinating, and keep your eyes fixed on the end goal.

through prayer and meditation. Studying, driving, and listening are activities that require mental focus. Yet prayer and meditation (which can be enhanced when sung) can produce the same, if not greater, responses in the body's ability to learn and improve memory. The nervous system produces electrical impulses in the form of alpha and beta waves in response to changes in our thoughts and mental activities. Alpha waves dominate when we daydream or feel drowsy, while the beta waves are characteristic of focused concentration, memory, and recall, which are enhanced when in a state of prayer and meditation. Beta waves are important for creating lasting change. Through prayer and meditation, we can break out of our negative thought patterns. Bad habits and addictions are broken when you practice demonstrating new behaviors and habits. The practice begins to override the old nature. While in this state of consciousness, we are not worrying about the future or mulling over the past but instead experiencing "mindfulness" or "being in the present moment." Mindfulness is similar to the state we are in when we drive down the highway, mesmerized by the road, forgetting what is going on around us. Olympic athletes describe this as the "Zone." Their concentration is so focused on the goal that distractions melt away.

During my early years of college at the University of Colorado, I ran cross country and track. My coach would take us out early on Sunday mornings for long runs averaging around 12 miles. I would start out thinking of the day's events, but then I would switch my focus to the rhythm of my breathing, and my concentration entered into a state of timelessness. Without realizing it, I had entered the "Zone," oblivious to my physical state, untethered by mental distractions. Running becomes painless while in this state of consciousness. By setting aside a daily time to "flow" into the Zone, you can enter into this portal, a state of joy, fulfillment, and gratitude.

Toxic Mindset Eraser

Once we become more practiced at mindfulness, it is possible to maintain calm, focused concentration even while enduring an unfavorable situation. To take this a step further, visual imagery can be used to reframe your reality through visualizing a healthier you or an abundant future. As you meditate and pray, focus your attention on the specific outcomes you want to see manifested in your life. Move around in that picture, making the image 3D and in full living color. Feel as if you are living and believing that picture of you. Return to this place of healing, this feeling of wholeness and wellness several times a day. Before long, you will bring into your experience what your heart has desired.

Envision the new you as a favorite memory already complete and manifested in your life. Draw a picture of this scene, or write a song, poem, or story about this new you! This practice retrains your subconscious mind to believe what you are writing, while your brain creates new neural pathways which, with practice, become your reality. Place the picture or poem on your fridge or the dashboard of your car. Gain the support of others by sharing your goals and soliciting their support and encouragement. This exercise allows you to erase deeply embedded destructive habits, replacing them with positive, self-nurturing behaviors. Soon your goals will be achieved and the imagery becomes your new reality.

EXERCISE 4: ENVISION THE REAL YOU

Position yourself in a comfortable, quiet area, free of distraction, for the next 15 minutes. Read the following instructions a few times before doing the exercise or you can record your voice reading the instructions and then it play it back.

Begin by taking a slow, deep breath, allowing your lungs to fill completely with air. Hold the breath for two to three seconds, then exhale slowly. Continue taking five to eight deep breaths, allowing yourself to relax a little deeper with each breath, imagining the tension melting away. Visualize your lungs completely filling up with life-giving oxygen. Be patient with yourself. When you notice that your mind has drifted off, gently bring your attention back to the breath, releasing any stressful thoughts and tension in your body. Once you are relaxed, tell yourself, "I am in a peaceful state of relaxation and health. Through the Creator of the Universe I am surrendering all my tension, frustration and resentments."

Become aware of any residual tension in your head, neck and shoulders. With each exhale, release the tension. Say to yourself, "I am now inviting in a peaceful state of love, self-acceptance, and a sound mind." Slowly breathe in and when you exhale, let any remaining tension go. Relax, and allow any negative thoughts or pictures from your day to drift away.

Now focus on your extremities, including your hands and feet. Take a deep breath in and when you exhale let any tension in these areas go. Do not hold stress; put your fingers in a relaxed state, palms facing up. Breathe and relax. Focus your attention on any tension in your legs and buttocks. Take a deep breath in and on the exhale release. Start to allow your entire body to melt into your surroundings. Continue deeply relaxing into the floor with each deep inhale and let all negative thoughts and stress go on the exhale. Now feel your feet and toes resting on the floor and allow any tension to leave your body. You are now prepared to enter into a state of deep meditation.

Now imagine yourself in a beautiful place--one that you find pleasing. Smell the pure crisp air and feel the warm breeze brush lightly against your skin. Picture a crystal clear lake, at the perfect temperature, and start to walk into the water. You feel a gentle caress from the healing water as you lay back and begin to float effortlessly. You feel clean and weightless. Now visualize your body at a healthy weight and completely disease-free. Your entire body is strong and beautiful. The feeling of the water against your skin has given you a sense of complete contentment. Your body is a sacred temple--all of your organs are fully functioning, working together as a harmonious whole.

Void of the sense of urgency that normally plagues you, your heart beats effortlessly. The sense of deep relaxation has engulfed you as you continue peacefully floating in the crystal clear water, your lungs taking in as much oxygen as they need. You are the caretaker of this beautiful vessel. You feel incredible.

Floating toward you is a basket filled with the choicest fruits. Choose one, and bite into the juicy sweetness. The fruit tastes so divine that it completely satisfies and nourishes every cell in your body.

Gently begin to come back into the moment. Feel the air against your skin. Hear the sounds of the room around you. Slowly begin to move your fingers and toes as you bring your conscious awareness into this space. Carry this sense of peace and contentment with you as you slowly open your eyes. You have developed a greater awareness of ownership over your body. You understand more clearly that every good and perfect choice you make will revive and heal every aspect of your body.

Tell yourself that your body is a gift from God and be thankful for it. You accept the Creator's principle that overeating and eating toxic foods poison your body. You desire only to give yourself foods that will protect and honor your body.

Now you see yourself emerging from the crystal pure water, overjoyed and refreshed. Notice how graceful and light your body moves and feels. You are aware of the power God has placed within you to be completely whole. When your intention is to have a joyful and healthy body, every step you take from this point forward has the ability to glorify and heal the body.

Repeat these words seven times over:

I love and respect myself.
I am thankful for this beautiful body and mind.
I must guard them.
Overeating is a poison.
I choose to honor my body.

As you ready yourself to leave this time of prayer and meditation, remind yourself to stay focused on the resolutions you have made. The more clearly you can visualize the you God created you to be, the greater success you will have in arriving at a stronger, more radiant, and more confident you.

Conclusion

If you only have time to read and apply one chapter of this book I pray it is this one. Lasting and effective change in your life can only come about if you first identify your self-limiting behavior, forgive yourself and/or those who have wronged you, dump your toxic habits and behaviors, even if they are just the distractions of a busy life, and then retrain your mind to believe you are full of joy and posses an abundant life. You may identify with the stories of my sister Alyssa or the Nazi camp survivor Viktor Frankl; or you may be on your own unique journey, searching for healing. Either way, I believe you can--and will--overcome your toxic mindset!

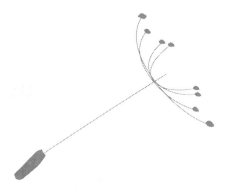

Drink and Shower with Purified Water-- Look and Feel Younger!

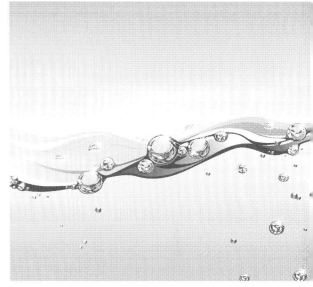

Take a moment to imagine just how important water is to us. You are standing on a sandy slope in the middle of the Sahara Desert. A hot, dry gust of wind buffets your emaciated body. The heat is heavy. A few grains of sand hit your face. Your tongue is thick and dry as you squint your eyes against the harsh sun to gaze into the distance. Is it real? Your mind plays tricks on you. You hope the wavering mirage of a small cluster of palms is real. Your feet sluggishly follow your brain's feeble command.

Your hope has been dashed time and again since your Saharan dune buggy finally sputtered to a halt thirsting for gas. You curse the sand storm that disoriented you from your guide several days before. Your skin is cracking, rough, and red, and the 130-degree heat is quickly wicking away the remaining moisture from your body. Your mind is delusional; you hear voices from all directions shouting your name. You focus. The palms still dance in the distant heat. You plod on. The sand gives way and engulfs your feet hungrily with each step. You try to swallow to make your throat comfortable, but your adam's apple is unwilling to respond. Your throat has become more swollen and tight as the hours have trickled away like the last of your water a day ago. Minutes pass, hours pass, and you are humbled to all fours. Crawling and pulling with the last of your efforts you reach the cool spring. Finally, salvation in the middle of a barren sandy wasteland.

The vibrant life of the soothing, smooth water dances down your burning throat. The water brings hope, brings life, and brings understanding about the source of life. Slowly the puffiness around your eyes decreases, your internal organs cool from their inflamed state, and after a few hours your mind can form complete thoughts. You become aware of the nearby birds and enjoy the melodic symphony of their voices. It is now easy to appreciate their joy as they happily frolic in the shallow pools cleaning their wings.

• • •

Besides the air you breathe, water is the next most essential element impacting for all physiological functions of your body, and it is impossible to live without it for more than three days. Long before you would die from starvation, you would die from dehydration, as the picture above illustrates.

Water constitutes approximately 70% of your body, 83% of your brain, 75% of your muscles, and 90% of your blood. Water affects every major function in your body, including transportation of nutrients and oxygen to your cells, regulating body temperature, cushioning your joints, controlling the metabolic rate of your biochemical reactions (e.g., fat burning, digestion, and blood sugar regulation), and the removal of bodily wastes. Water reduces your risk of certain cancers, boosts mental performance, aids in weight loss, improves digestion, helps the body recover from physical injuries, and aids in the detoxification of impurities within the body.

Without proper hydration from water some of the most common symptoms are: headaches, tiredness, lack of energy, fogginess or unclear thoughts, acne and skin issues, strong body odor, mood changes, and irritability, to name a few. In a nutshell, pure water carries life to our cells in order for our body to live optimally. But not all water is healthy and not all areas of the world have adequate water supplies. Choosing the right source of water is imperative for enhancing your health and ridding your body of disease.

> Water constitutes approximately 70% of your body, 83% of your brain, 75% of your muscles, and 90% of your blood.

In the U.S., we have many options for where to get our water. In this chapter, we will examine the dangers found lurking in tap water as well as some surprising truths about bottled, distilled, and reverse osmosis water. Just because it's in a plastic bottle doesn't mean your water is safe for you! And finally, we will discover where to find the best source of pure, healthy water.

The small doses of lethal toxins ingested when consuming impure water can manifest over time in life-threatening illnesses and diseases such as:

• **High blood pressure**	• **Joint aches**	• **Obesity**	• **Lymphoma**
• **High cholesterol**	• **Fatigue**	• **Headaches**	• **Angina**
• **Thyroid disorders**	• **Hypertension**	• **Allergies**	• **Heartburn**
• **Liver disease**	• **Edema**	• **Depression**	• **Back pain**
• **Constipation**	• **Acne**	• **Anxiety**	• **Colitis**
• **Autoimmune diseases**	• **Lupus**	• **Type 2 diabetes**	• **Cancer**
• **Fibromyalgia pain**	• **Migraines**	• **Parkinson's disease**	• **And many more!**
• **Sleep disorders**	• **Sinusitis**	• **Alzheimer's**	

And, to make matters worse, instead of hydrating with healing water, people often take drugs for these problems that further imbalance their bodies. There are thousands of articles and studies written in journals and newspapers and posted on websites to disseminate information on the hazardous potential of contaminants in municipal (tap) water. We will only touch on a couple of areas, with our focus on chlorine and fluoride and how they promote cancer development and disrupt hormones.

Chlorine

It is widely accepted that tap water contains chlorine, a powerful oxidizer that not only kills microorganisms but also oxidizes and attacks the DNA in all living matter. You and I are living matter. When our very DNA is attacked, it can cause damage that will eventually result in permanent cellular alteration which can lead to premature aging and cancer. In addition, chlorine reacts with organic material in our water to produce a family of compounds known as chlorination byproducts and trihalomethanes. These compounds have been directly linked to the long-term development of cancer in very low concentrations.[1] The U.S. Council of Environmental Quality states that, "Cancer risk among people drinking chlorinated water is 93% higher than among those whose water does not contain chlorine." And Francis T. Mayo, Director of Municipal Environmental Research Laboratory, said, "Known carcinogens are found in drinking water as a direct consequence of the practice of chlorination. Using chlorine has been a long established pubic health practice for the disinfection of drinking water." Dr. Riddle from the Kemysts Laboratory states, "Scientific studies have linked chlorine and chlorination by-products to cancer of the bladder, liver, stomach, rectum, and colon, as well as heart disease, atherosclerosis (hardening of the arteries), anemia, high blood pressure, and allergic reactions. There is also evidence that shows that chlorine can destroy protein in our body and cause adverse effects on skin and hair."[2]

If you're concerned about drinking chlorinated water, you should be twice as concerned about showering in it. One study found that six to 100 times more toxins can be absorbed by the skin and by breathing the steam and air around unfiltered showers than drinking it! In fact, the chlorine exposure from one shower is equal to an entire day's amount of drinking the same water. This is alarming knowing that over 600% of toxins are absorbed into your open pores in a hot shower (in comparison to drinking that same water all day long)![3] The Environmental Protection Agency now reports that individuals who drink and bathe in chlorinated surface waters have a 50% greater likelihood of getting cancer in their lifetime.[4] So by drinking pure, filtered water you are only solving half the problem.

Here's a short list of pollutants typically found in unfiltered shower and drinking water (if you get your water from a private well, all of these contaminants may be present except for the chlorination byproducts):[5,6,7,8,9]

- Fecal matter
- Viruses
- Parasite
- Bacteria
- Fungus
- Pesticides
- Heavy metals
- Radioactive compounds

- Petrochemicals
- Chlorine/chloramines
- Fluoride
- Pharmaceutical drugs (including narcotics, birth control, antibiotics, anti-depressants)

- Hormone blockers
- Cancer-causing nitrates
- Estrogens
- Volatile Organic Compounds (VOC's)
- Trihalomethanes (THM's)
- Bad taste, odors, and more!

Fluoride

Fluoride is equally as toxic to our hormone and thyroid functions as any other source in water. Problems caused by fluoride include dental fluorosis (a disease of the teeth), weakening of bones, bone loss, bone cancer, and kidney problems. The National Research Council (NRC) warns that ingestion of only .01-.03 mg/kg per day of fluoride, which is easily achieved by drinking fluoridated water, can severely inhibit proper thyroid and hormone function.[10]

Healthy hormone levels help to balance your mood, immune system, weight, and energy in conjunction with a balanced lifestyle. So when toxins raise your natural hormone levels, diseases and cancer manifest rapidly. In 2007, the Seattle Times published an article about male fish swimming in Seattle's Elliott Bay carrying a protein usually found only in female fish with developing eggs. These "feminized" fish, first discovered in the late 90's, are the victims of chemicals in the water—chemicals from human birth-control pills, hormone-replacement therapy drugs, plastic bottles, and makeup, which ended up in the water from septic tanks or leaking sewer pipes. The reproductive systems of the males were not the only ones affected; female fish were producing

You may want to research further what contaminants do to you. Check out the National Primary Drinking Water Standards: **www.water-research.net/ standards.htm**. If you are on a public water system, you can call the water utility company and request a copy of the utility's most recent Consumer Confidence Report. Learn more at **www.fluoridealert.org**.

eggs several months after their usual spawning seasons and reaching sexual maturity at a younger age, according to researchers at the Northwest Fisheries Science Center. And these startling discoveries are not limited to Washington; they are now occurring all over the country in states like California, Colorado, and Nevada.[11] If fish are experiencing changes, you can bet that humans are experiencing the same.

And they are. One segment of the population affected is young girls who are entering puberty at extremely early ages. In 1973, the average age for puberty 12.8 years. In 1997, a landmark study written by Marcia Herman-Giddens, adjunct professor at the School of Public Health at the University of North Carolina-Chapel Hill, found that among 17,000 girls in North Carolina, almost half of blacks and 15% of whites had begun breast development by age eight. And now, researchers at Oregon Health and Science University's Primate Research Center are trying to figure out why some girls as young as four or five are entering puberty.[12] Until ten years ago, breast development at age eight was considered an abnormal event that should be investigated by an endocrinologist. Just because this is happening more frequently does not mean this is normal--it is NOT normal! It is direct result of the fluoride and other toxins in our drinking water and in the standard American diet.

In order to prevent future and current health-related issues, you must eliminate as many sources of toxicity in your life as possible! Clearly, public water supplies must be avoided for optimal health. But what about alternatives such as Reverse Osmosis and distilled water? Reverse Osmosis or RO strips the water of all its minerals in the process of trying to purify the water. This means that the water is void of the essential trace minerals you should be absorbing (up to 90% or your trace minerals come from the water you drink). RO also removes the alkaline mineral constituents of water, thus producing acidic water. If dead and void water is put in your body it will steal minerals from your body to become balanced.

Not only is it not healthy, but RO also wastes up to three gallons of water just to make one gallon of "purified" water. This also increases the costs of filter replacement and maintenance due to the encrustation or scaling of minerals on the membrane. RO is not a cost-effective or safe alternative as a purified water source.

As for distilled water, distillation also produces acidic mineral-free water and does not remove chlorine, chlorine byproducts, or VOC's. Eighty percent of the water is discarded with the contaminants, wasting up to FIVE gallons for every one gallon of purified water produced! It is, however, great for use during a cleansing process or for laboratory work. Thus, distilled water is not a cost-effective or safe alternative water source, either.

Many health institutes, doctors, sports and fitness centers, and clinics around the world are now recommending using filtration systems that purify and enhance your water while removing 99.9999% of contaminants.

Proper filtration adds essential trace minerals that naturally occur in spring water to increase your energetic and biological functions. Water treated with proper filtration has a natural resistance to the growth of harmful bacteria and fungi. It also increases the rate of hydration of the skin and tissues, thus accelerating the rate of nutrient absorption into the bloodstream. Users have reported a noticeable increase of energy in all areas of health including improved digestion, elimination, mental clarity, and weight loss. In Japan many doctors routinely prescribe the filtered water to their patients to aid the body in fighting specific chronic conditions.

Look for filtered water that has the ability to:

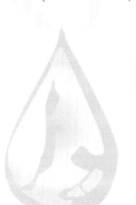

- Hydrate instantaneously
- Enhance the taste of water and food
- Increase vitality and energy
- Lower blood pressure and cholesterol
- Greatly decrease your chance of kidney stones and cancers
- Increase absorption of vitamins and minerals
- Balance the pH of blood and saliva, providing an alkalinizing effect
- Regulate your appetite when you drink water before a meal
- Support the growth of healthy bacteria
- Hydrate and plump skin with its high silica content, as well as improve overall skin health if you have problems with eczema, psoriasis, acne, etc.
- Provide natural minerals and antioxidants
- Accelerate your body's removal of waste by-products (from exercise, metabolism and the environment)
- Make you retain less water
- Save you money
- Conserve energy
- Make your home safer

Properly filtered water removes:

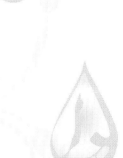

- Chlorine
- Heavy metals
- Fungus, mold, and feces
- Radioactive contaminants, petrochemicals

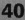

- Fluoride (it converts fluoride into calcium fluorite)
- Anaerobic bacteria
- Existing calcium and aragonite deposits
- Hormones and estrogens
- Pesticides and herbicides
- Plastic by-products
- Cancer-causing nitrates
- Pharmaceutical drugs (including narcotics, birth control, antibiotics, antidepressants and the like)
- Viruses

ACTION STEP:

Immediately start cutting out beverages like soda, coffee, black tea, and carbonated beverages that dehydrate and cause further oxidative stress in your body. Make the decision to stop drinking and bathing in toxic, disease-promoting waters. As soon as you can, replace all the water sources in your home with a filtration water unit. Use a shower filter that hydrates, protects, nourishes, and heals your body from illness, you will notice an immediate improvement to the firmness of your skin, health and energy levels. To start, drink a minimum of 64 ounces (8 8-ounce glasses) of properly filtered water a day and take one shower in filtered shower-water to improve circulation and the items listed above.

A good way for you to calculate how much water to drink is by your body weight; for every pound you weigh you are to have _ ounce of water per day. Or divide your body weight by two and drink that many ounces of water a day. For example, if you weigh 130 pounds you should drink approximately 64 ounces of water each day. You can calculate how much water your body weight needs at www.bottledwater.org/content/hydration-calculator.

Another thing to keep in mind is WHEN to drink. Make sure you are drinking water at the proper time to avoid diluting your stomach acids. This can impair assimilation of nutrients and cause malabsorption problems.

Best times to drink water:

When you wake up (20 oz.)
20 minutes before breakfast
Midmorning
20 minutes before lunch
Midafternoon
20 minutes before dinner
2 hours after dinner

With the way we live in America, it is not surprising that most of us never get enough water. Lemonade, iced tea, coffee, soda, or other liquids are not considered water. In fact, it has been shown that you need to drink eight glasses of water to balance out your body's pH from one can of cola. You cannot deny your body water or it will die! Drink purified water and, if you don't like the taste of water initially, jazz it up with the juice of a fresh lemon, lime, or cucumber. If you aren't used to drinking this much water it may take a couple weeks for your body to balance out. You may need to use the restroom more often, but please do not look at this as an inconvenience. Your body will finally be able to detoxify and carry away the waste sediment that has built up over time. Your kidneys and other organs are designed to cleanse until you are cleaned up, and then your thirsting cells will finally be hydrated and remain healthy and happy.

Endnotes

1 Carlo, George L. *Cancer Incidence and Trihalomethane Concentrations in the Public Drinking Water System.* American Journal of Public Health, Vol. 74, No. 5, 479-484, 1984.

2 http://holecomedispa.com/shower_filter_info.html

3 Anderson, Ian. *Showers Pose a Risk to Health.* New Scientist,September 18, 1986.

4 *Organic Chemical Contaminants in Drinking Water and Cancer.* American Journal of Epidemiology, Vol. 110, 420, 1979.

5 Richman, M. *Water Pollution.* Wastewater, Vol. 5, No. 2, 24-29, 1997.

6 http://www.water-research.net/helpguide.htm

7 *Probe: Pharmaceuticals In Drinking Water.* March 10, 2008; accessed Dec. 16, 2009, http://www.cbsnews.com/stories/2008/03/10/health/main3920454.shtml

8 McKone, Thomas E. *Human exposure to volatile organic compounds in household tap water: the indoor inhalation pathway.* Environ. Sci. Techno., Vol. 21, No. 12, 1194-1201, Dec. 1987.

9 Scully, Frank E., Jr. *Proteins in natural waters and their relation to the formation of chlorinated organics during water disinfection.* Environ. Sci. Technol., Vol. 22, No. 5, 537-542, May 1988.

10 Huff, Ethan. *Fluoride Causes Cancer and Hormone Disruption.* Dec. 9, 2009; accessed Dec. 16, 2009, http://www.ethiopianreview.com/health/26160

11 Cornwall, Warren and Ervin, Keith. *Hormonal chemicals may be imperiling fish.* April 1, 2007; accessed Dec. 16, 2009, http://seattletimes.nwsource.com/html/localnews/2003645892_hormone01m.html

12 Miles, Christine. "Puberty Hitting Girls At Younger Age." Jan.30, 2002; accessed Dec. 16, 2009, http://www.freerepublic.com/focus/fr/618790/posts

Cleanse The Body--Flush Away Toxins

1. Total Body Cleanse--For Maximum Cleaning
2. Mild Total Body Cleanse--Short and Sweet!
3. Easy Does It Liver Cleanse
4. One Day Gallstone Purge

An Overview of Cleansing

Since Biblical times, people have been fasting and cleansing for many reasons including better health, disease recovery, spiritual enlightenment, and political protest. However, in our day and age the most people are not educated on the health benefits fasting and cleansing can provide. Before we can create healthy bodies and minds we must substitute toxic foods with foods high in nutritional value. But before doing that, it is best to allow the body to heal itself through a process of cleansing. This will raise the "life" of the cells, changing them from magnets for disease to strong guardians of health. The person with a toxin-free body and a sound mind is the person unaffected by epidemics.

Cleansing is an excellent way to rid the body of toxicities caused by pesticides, chemicals, parasites, artificial flavors and colors, preservatives, rancid oils, and pollutants that are stored in various organs, cells, and in fat tissue. Symptoms of toxic overload include digestive problems, joint pain, headaches, low energy, allergic reactions, asthma, allergies, anxiety, depression, mental confusion, and disease. Cleansing is an opportunity for new beginnings--to renew, regroup, and recuperate lost energy and health. For optimal health, a cleanse is recommended twice a year—once in the spring and once in the fall, as these are the optimal times for releasing toxins.

A typical body cleanse involves fasting from all solid foods, drinking fresh fruit and vegetable juices, taking specific supplements, performing enemas or having colonics, and doing minimal exercises. It is also advisable to spend as much time as possible resting.

If you have never done a cleanse before, it may seem like a challenge. However, the type of cleanse we suggest to our first time clients, the Mild Total Body Cleanse, is a better fit for most lifestyles. Mild cleansing is of great benefit to the novice who wants to experience the benefits of cleansing with minimal ingredients. Your first experience sets the stage for all other detox plans you do in the future. So the better the experience and completion of the mild cleanse, the longer the results. Again, it is suggested that you do a detox two times a year, once in the spring and the other in the fall. If you have already done some cleanses, or are dealing with a serious illness or allergies, then you will want to complete the full Total Body Cleanse.

If you have been diagnosed with an illness and/or are taking prescription medications, cleansing should be done under the direct supervision of a health practitioner. During the cleanse be aware that you may experience nausea, headaches, dizziness, extreme hunger, and feverish-like chills. While this does not happen to everyone, it is the body's reaction to toxic overload.

When planning a cleanse, start by preparing your body for the process. Three days prior to beginning, eat only fresh and raw vegetables, fruits, and seeds. During the cleanse, drink distilled water if possible as this helps reduce hunger pains; the molecules of purified, spring, or tap water actually cause the body to search for food. However, it is permissible to drink spring water if you prefer. During the cleanse you will experience highs and lows, so be gracious to yourself. Spend time stretching and breathing deeply throughout the day. Sun bathe if possible for 15-20 minutes per day. Soak in an Epsom salt bath each evening. These activities will help to regenerate your cells as you cleanse them.

For the beginner, enemas may be a stumbling block. However, they do maximize the amount of toxins that are removed from the body and aid in the release of gallstones. If you do not feel comfortable performing enemas, you can either omit them or look into hiring a colon hydro therapist. Specific instructions for the enemas recommended for the Total Body Cleanse are provided later in this chapter.

When you have completed your cleanse, allow two to three days' transition to let your colon relearn to digest whole foods. If you eat too much too soon, the body will experience an overload and toxins will again start accumulating from undigested food.

Remember, your mind is a powerful tool; it can hinder or help you cleanse. So keep a positive mental attitude, read uplifting books, pray, meditate, stretch, lie in the sun, take Epsom salt baths, and do moderate activity while you cleanse.

1. TOTAL BODY CLEANSE--FOR MAXIMUM CLEANING

Warning: Seek the help of your health care provider before starting any cleanse. The three or seven-day Total Body Cleanse is not advised for pregnant or lactating women or for anyone with a serious illness. It is done at your own risk. Some people have reported headaches, nausea, dizziness, and fatigue with this cleanse. Occasionally the body is more toxic than it appears and can cause unforeseen problems. You may or may not experience these symptoms, depending on your overall health. If you have had your gallbladder removed, skip the olive oil drinks and perform only the water enemas. Proceed at your own risk.

It is suggested to drink the amount listed below in the daily schedule. However, if you feel like you are stuffing yourself with liquids, reduce the daily amount to suit your physical needs. I have found in my own practice that some who have had gallbladders removed tend to feel stuffed using the apple juice mixture. If you have had your gallbladder removed you can replace half of the apple juice mixture with fresh cantaloupe juice. For example, replace 2 ½ cups of diluted apple juice with 2 ½ cups of diluted canteloupe juice.

Instructions for the Total Body Cleanse are provided for both three days and seven days on the pages following this overview. The longer you do the cleanse the longer lasting the results will be. This cleanse helps to:
- Rid the liver of toxic debris and excess bile
- Clear gallstones
- Remove compacted fecal matter in the colon
- Clean cells
- Purify the blood from bacteria, fungus, and viruses
- Repair injured tissues (tendons, organs, muscles, etc.)

SUPPLEMENTS AND FOODS NEEDED FOR 3-DAY TOTAL BODY CLEANSE

(Amounts for 7-day cleanse are in parenthesis)
- 1 (2) jar of Barley Greens (AIM™) (or fresh wheat grass juice)
- 5-7 (10-15) pounds organic carrots for juicing
- 1 jar of Herbal Fiberblend (by AIM™)
- 6 (12) ounces ground chia seed or ground psyllium husks

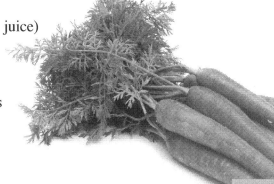

- Probiotics (New Chapter™)
- Fresh garlic
- 1 (2) bag of organic apples for juicing *or*
  1 (2) gallon organic apple juice
- 4 (6) organic grapefruits
- 16 (20) ounces extra virgin olive oil
- 8 (14) gallons distilled water
- Organic clove powder
- 1 container Epsom salts
- 1 enema bag (called water bag or douche bag)
- 1 bag organic coffee grounds

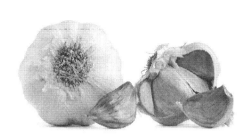

  ---Optional---
- 5-6 organic lemons
- Aussie Sea Minerals/Supa Boost

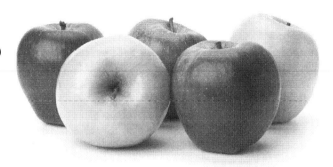

ADVICE ABOUT PURCHASING THE INGREDIENTS:

- AIM™ Products: Barley Life, Herbal Fiberblend, and Just Carrots can be ordered through the AIM™ company. Call toll free at 1-800-456-2462 and give them my referral number, #591683, to receive a member discount.
- Order Aussie Sea Minerals (optional) at www.foodbeautiful.com.
- If you prefer garlic pills to fresh garlic, it is best to purchase the Liquid Kyolic™ rather than garlic capsules to save your stomach the work of breaking down gelatin capsules during the cleanse.
- Other supplements and organic produce can be purchased from Whole Foods®, Wild Oats®, Vitamin Cottage™, Trader Joe's®, online, or at your local health food store. Make sure to purchase only organic food products as you do not want to add additional stress on the body from pesticides while you are cleansing.

It is a wise idea to read through the information about enemas and all the cleanse instructions provided on the following pages a couple of times before starting. This will help you better understand the process.

PLANNING YOUR CLEANSE:

Planning ahead makes all the difference. Here are some ideas. If you generally work during the week and have weekends off, you can plan a 3-day cleanse (which actually takes 3 ½ days) starting on a Thursday. That way the days you'll be doing three enemas will fall on Saturday and Sunday. For the 7-day fast, starting on a Sunday will put the three enema days on Friday, Saturday, and Sunday. This allows your body optimal rest during the enema days.

GENERAL INFORMATION ABOUT ENEMAS:

In this modern, toxic world it's becoming a simple fact of life that our colon is the sewer system of the body. Enemas clear out compacted fecal matter, pesticides, and other pollutants taken in from our air, water, and food. The liver and other organs also release stored toxins into the colon. Water enemas clear these toxins. The coffee/lemon juice/hyssop tea mixture stimulates the release of toxic liver bile and stored gallstones in the gallbladder. Once you have completed either the 3-day or 7-day cleanse with the suggested enemas, you will have accomplished an internal cleanse of your organs and cells. Detailed instructions about enema procedures are provided below.

3-DAY CLEANSE:

For the first and second day of this cleanse do one water enema upon arising. A second water enema in the mid- to late-afternoon is optional to remove excess toxins that may cause discomfort, such as extreme headaches, dizziness, and nausea. On the third and fourth days do these three enemas each morning upon arising:

1) Water
2) Coffee/lemon juice/hyssop tea
3) Probiotic

Set aside two hours in the morning to complete the three enemas on each of these days. They are to be done back to back, with time in between for complete evacuation. You may pass gallstones, often the size and color of peas, through the stool during these days. Unlike passing a stone through the urine, gallstones are painless.

7-DAY CLEANSE:

For the first five days of this cleanse do one water enema upon arising. A second water enema in the mid- to late-afternoon is optional to remove excess toxins that may cause discomfort, such as extreme headaches, dizziness, and nausea. On the sixth, seventh, and eighth, days do three enemas each morning upon arising:

1) Water

2) Coffee/lemon juice/hyssop tea

3) Probiotic

Set aside two hours in the morning to complete the three enemas on each of these days. They are to be done back to back, with time in between for complete evacuation. You may pass gallstones, often the size and color of peas, through the stool during these days. Unlike passing a stone through the urine, gallstones are painless.

Note: Complete instructions for each type of enema are provided below.

ENEMA INSTRUCTIONS:

Enema bags can be purchased at any drug store. They consist of a 2-quart capacity rubber bag, a hose, and a nozzle. The bag is filled with liquid and hung above the body, close enough for the hose to reach the rectum. The nozzle is inserted into the rectum. A valve on the hose allows the user to control the flow of liquid into the colon. An enema involves putting liquids into your colon, holding the liquid for a period of time and then evacuating the liquids into a toilet. Evacuation can take from 2 to 15 minutes for each enema. Just be patient.

Make sure to read and follow the instructions provided with the enema bag you are using.

TYPES OF ENEMAS:

- **Distilled Water Enema**: Two quarts of distilled water, warmed to 98°F in your enema bag.

- **Organic Coffee Enema:** Combine one quart of water and 4-6 tablespoons of organic coffee and run it through a drip coffee maker. If you don't have a coffee maker, boil the ground coffee in the water for 15 minutes. Strain through a coffee filter or cheese cloth to remove the grounds. Dilute the prepared coffee with one quart of distilled water. Warm the diluted coffee to 98°F and pour into the enema bag for use.

- **Probiotic Enema:** A coffee enema must be followed by a probiotic enema to reestablish healthy intestinal flora, which is killed by the coffee. Empty two probiotic capsules into two quarts of warmed distilled (98°F) water and fill the enema bag.

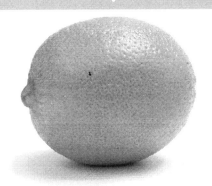

Note: If you're sensitive to caffeinated coffee, substitute with organic decaffeinated coffee, lemon juice, or hyssop tea as explained below.

- **Lemon Juice Enema:** Add the juice of ½ lemon to two quarts of warmed (98°F) distilled water. Pour into an enema bag for use.

- **Hyssop Tea Enema:** Add eight teaspoons of loose hyssop herb to one quart of water. Bring to a boil and allow to steep for 20 minutes. Remove the hyssop herb by straining the tea through cheesecloth. Dilute the quart of tea with one quart of distilled water, heat to 98°F, and pour into an enema bag for use.

ENEMA PROCEDURE:

Use an enema bag with a rectal tube or a Faultless® brand fountain syringe. If you use a fountain syringe, it is important to use the douche nozzle, which is long enough to extend beyond the nerve endings in the rectum. Lubricate the rectal tube or douche nozzle with KY® jelly or olive oil. DO NOT use petroleum jelly or any other petroleum product including mineral oil, which will destroy the vitamins and minerals in the colon. Have a small bowl of water containing a disinfectant solution (soap and water) available in which to place the nozzle following the enema procedure.

Prepare a comfortable place to lie on the bathroom floor with towels and pillows. Position the enema bag no higher than 20 inches above the hips; for example, hanging from the doorknob. Lie on your back and insert the lubricated tube or douche tip into the rectum. Release the clamp on the hose to allow the solution to enter the colon slowly. When pressure builds, clamp the flow and lay on your right side (Note: It is okay to stay lying on your back if that is more comfortable). Massage your abdomen with a small handful amount of olive oil, moving left to right in line of the colon (in an upside down U shape) until you feel more comfortable. When the pressure subsides, resume until all the solution has been used. Never let the pressure get intolerable. Remove the nozzle, hold the solution in the rectum for 7-10 minutes and evacuate it into the toilet. If you can't hold in the liquid that long you may evacuate sooner. After you have held the liquid in for 7-10 minutes, you can speed up the evacuation of fluids from the colon by massaging the colon from right to left. Clean the nozzle in the soap and water. For the second and third enemas, lie on alternate sides, or on your back when massaging the abdomen. Always try to massage following the line of the colon from left to right when you are doing the enema. It is ideal to retain the coffee enema for a full 15 minutes before evacuating. This allows the coffee enough time to do its job. After the coffee enema you will finish up with the probiotics enema.

Day 1 (of 3-Day Cleanse) / Day 1-4 (of 7-Day Cleanse)

Upon Arising

Drink 1-2 tablespoons Barley Life mixed with 6-8 ounces water *or* drink 3 ounces freshly juiced wheat grass.

Wait 30-45 minutes, then drink 2 tablespoons olive oil mixed in 4 ounces freshly squeezed grapefruit juice or lemon juice. If possible go back to bed and lay on your right side with your right knee to your chest for 20 minutes.

(Caution: If your gallbladder has been removed, skip the olive oil)

Complete 1 distilled water enema.

Start of the Day

Drink 2 teaspoons Herbal Fiberblend and 1 ½ teaspoons ground chia seed mixed with 8 ounces fresh apple juice and 4 ounces distilled water. About 30 minutes later, drink the first of five additional cups of 8 ounces apple juice with 4 ounces water.

Finish all five cups before midafternoon.

Tip: Pre-mix the entire portion for the day

Optional: Add the juice of one lemon to the five cups of apple juice for flavor.

Optional: Have 1 teaspoon Sea Minerals in 4 oz of juice.

Diabetics: Have one scoop of protein powder with 2 of the five servings.

Mid to Late Afternoon

Mix 1 tablespoon Just Carrots in 10 ounces of water with 1 teaspoon Barley Life powder and ½ teaspoon Liquid Kyolic™ garlic with each drink. Drink five cups of this before 8 p.m.
-OR-
Mix 7 ounces fresh carrot juice with 3 ounces distilled water. Add 1 teaspoon Barley Life powder and ½ teaspoon Liquid Kyolic™ garlic with each drink. Drink five cups of this before 8 p.m.

Around 7 p.m. mix 2 teaspoons Herbal Fiberblend and 2 teaspoons ground chia seed with one of the servings of the carrot juice mixture.

Tip: Pre-mix the entire portions for the day.

Optional: Complete 1 distilled water enema.

Day 1 (of 3-Day Cleanse) / Day 1-4 (of 7-Day Cleanse)

Prior to Bed

Drink 1 tablespoon Barley Life mixed with 4 ounces distilled water or 3 ounces freshly juiced wheat grass.

Note: Staying hydrated is important so drink plenty of additional distilled or purified water throughout the cleanse. Never feel as though you need to stuff down that last 8 ounce glass of juice. It is okay if you cannot finish all the servings of juices. Each individual has different caloric needs.

Day 2 (of 3-Day Cleanse) / Day 5 (of 7-Day Cleanse)

Upon Arising

Drink an 8-ounce glass of distilled water containing 1-2 tablespoons of Epsom salts.

30-45 minutes later drink 2 tablespoons Barley Life mixed with 8 ounces water or 3 ounces fresh-juiced wheat grass.

20 minutes later drink 2 tablespoons olive oil mixed in 4 ounces freshly squeezed grapefruit or lemon juice. If possible go back to bed and lay on your right side with your right knee to your chest for 20 minutes.

Complete 1 distilled water enema.

Start of the Day

Mix 2 teaspoons Herbal Fiberblend and ½ teaspoon ground chia seed with 8 ounces fresh apple juice and 4 ounces distilled water.

About 30 minutes later, drink the first of five additional cups of 8 ounces apple juice with 4 ounces water. Finish all five cups before mid-afternoon.

Optional: Add the juice of one lemon to the five cups of apple juice for flavor.

Optional: Have 1 teaspoon Sea Minerals in 4 oz of juice.

Day 2 (of 3-Day Cleanse) / Day 5 (of 7-Day Cleanse)

Mid Afternoon

Mix 1 tablespoon Just Carrots in 10 ounces of water with 1 teaspoon Barley Life powder and ½ teaspoon Liquid Kyolic™ garlic with each drink. Drink five cups of this before 8 p.m.
-OR-
Mix 7 ounces fresh carrot juice with 3 ounces distilled water. Add 1 teaspoon Barley Life powder and ½ teaspoon Liquid Kyolic™ garlic with each drink. Drink five cups of this before 8 p.m.

Tip: Pre-mix the entire portion for the day.

Late Afternoon

Between 5 -6 p.m. Combine 8 ounces of warm distilled water with 1-2 tablespoons Epsom salts. Note: this step is crucial to the effectiveness of the cleanse.

Around 7 p.m. mix 2 teaspoons Herbal Fiberblend and 1 ½ teaspoons ground chia seed with 8 ounces carrot juice and 4 ounces water.

Optional: Complete 1 distilled water enema.

Prior to Bed

Drink 4 ounces cold pressed, extra virgin olive oil with 4 ounces fresh-juiced grapefruit or lemon juice and ¼ to ½ teaspoon clove powder (to prevent nausea during the night).

Go to bed immediately and lay on your right side with your right knee to your chest for 20 minutes.

(Caution: if your gallbladder has been removed, skip the olive oil.)

Important reminder: Drink plenty of additional distilled or purified water throughout the cleanse.

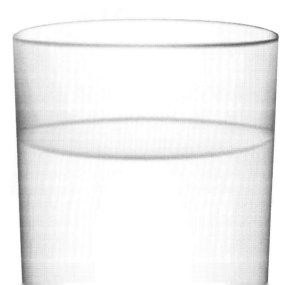

Day 3 (of 3-Day Cleanse) / Day 6-7 (of 7-Day Cleanse)

Upon Rising

Drink an 8-ounce glass of distilled water containing 1-2 tablespoons of Epsom salts.

30-45 minutes later drink 2 tablespoons Barley Life mixed with 8 ounces water or 3 ounces fresh-juiced wheat grass.

Immediately following, complete 3 enemas (see enema directions):
1. Distilled water
2. Coffee (or lemon juice)
3. Probiotics

Note: Allow a total of 2 hours to complete the 3 enemas. Wait 15 minutes for evacuation between each enema.

Start of the Day

Mix 2 teaspoons Herbal Fiberblend with 1 ½ teaspoons ground chia seed with 8 ounces fresh apple juice and 4 ounces distilled water.

About 30 minutes later, drink the first of five additional cups of 8 ounces apple juice with 4 ounces water. Finish all five cups before mid-afternoon.

Optional: Add the juice of one lemon to the five cups of apple juice for flavor.

Optional: Have 1 teaspoon Sea Minerals in 4 ounces of juice.

Mid Afternoon

Mix 1 tablespoon Just Carrots in 10 ounces of water with 1 teaspoon Barley Life powder and ½ teaspoon Liquid Kyolic™ garlic with each drink. Drink five cups of this before 8 p.m.
-OR-
Mix 7 ounces fresh carrot juice with 3 ounces distilled water. Add 1 teaspoon Barley Life powder and ½ teaspoon Liquid Kyolic™ garlic with each drink. Drink five cups of this before 8 p.m.

Tip: Pre-mix the entire portion for the day.

Late Afternoon

Between 5-6 p.m. Combine 8 ounces of warm distilled water with 1-2 tablespoons Epsom salts. Note: This step is crucial to the effectiveness of the cleanse.

Around 7 p.m. mix 2 teaspoons Herbal Fiberblend and 1 ½ teaspoons ground chia seed with 8 ounces carrot juice and 4 ounces water.

Day 3 (of 3-Day Cleanse) / Day 6-7 (of 7-Day Cleanse)

Prior to Bed

Drink 4 ounces cold pressed, extra virgin olive oil with 4 ounces fresh-juiced grapefruit or lemon juice and ¼ to ½ teaspoon clove powder (to prevent nausea during the night).

Go to bed immediately and lay on your right side with your right knee to your chest for 20 minutes.

Caution: if your gallbladder has been removed, skip the olive oil.

Important reminder: Drink plenty of additional distilled or purified water throughout the cleanse.

TRANSITIONING BACK TO FOOD
Day 4 (of 3-Day Cleanse) / Day 8 (of 7-Day Cleanse)

Upon Arising

Drink 2 tablespoons Barley Life mixed with 8 ounces water or 3 ounces freshly juiced wheat grass.

Immediately following, complete 3 enemas
(see enema directions):
1. Distilled water
2. Coffee (or lemon juice)
3. Probiotics

Note: Allow a total of 2 hours to complete the 3 enemas. Wait 15 minutes for evacuation between each enema.

Start of the Day

Mix 2 teaspoons Herbal Fiberblend and 1 ½ teaspoons ground chia seed mixed with 8 ounces fresh apple juice and 4 ounces distilled water.

20 minutes later have 1 grapefruit or apple.

Wait 20 minutes and have 10 ounces apple juice mixed with 6 ounces water.

Noon/Mid-Afternoon

Noon: Eat 1-2 pieces organic fresh fruit (grapefruit, mango, apple, peach, or pear). No bananas!

Mid-afternoon: Eat 1 cup steamed vegetables and vegetable broth soup.

TRANSITIONING BACK TO FOOD
Day 4 (of 3-Day Cleanse) / Day 8 (of 7-Day Cleanse)

Dinner
Light dinner: 1-2 cup steamed vegetables and vegetable broth, along with 5-10 brown rice crackers or ½ cup brown rice.   *Note: Make sure to chew your food slowly and thoroughly.*   The following day resume a normal diet, following the Food Beautiful Principles of Food Combining and Eat Healing Foods.

Important reminder: Drink plenty of additional spring or purified water throughout the cleanse. Do not use any more distilled water after the cleanse.

TRANSITIONING BACK TO FOOD
Day 9-10 (of 7-Day Cleanse)

Start of the Day
Mix 2 teaspoons Herbal Fiberblend and 1 ½ teaspoons ground chia seed with 8 ounces fresh apple juice and 4 ounces distilled water.   Eat 1-2 pieces organic fresh fruit (grapefruit, mango, apple, peach, or pear). No bananas!

Noon/Mid-Afternoon
Noon: Raw or steamed vegetable salad with ½ avocado and ½ cup beans of choice. Add 1 tablespoon coconut or olive oil into your dressing.   **Mid-afternoon:** Eat 1 apple with a handful of soaked almonds

Noon/Mid-Afternoon
Noon: Eat 1-2 pieces organic fresh fruit (grapefruit, mango, apple, peach, or pear). No bananas!   **Mid-afternoon:** Eat 1 cup steamed vegetables and vegetable broth soup.

2. MILD TOTAL BODY CLEANSE--SHORT AND SWEET!

Do this cleanse for 5-7 days as the purpose of this cleanse is to remove the toxins within your cells and allow weak organs and tissues to begin healing. This cleanse should be done before undertaking any new lifestyle/diet change. If you feel like it is to difficult to have only the lemonade all day long, than have brown rice and steamed vegetables in the evening and resume the cleansing cocktail during the day.

NOTE: Do not take supplements on this cleanse; allow your body to rest from any supplements or herbs. A good indication the cleanse is near completion is when a formerly fuzzy coated tongue becomes clear and pink looking again. If you are on prescription drugs consult your physician before starting any cleanse. Distilled water is used during this cleanse as it helps to draw out more toxins in the body while suppressing the appetite.

MILD TOTAL BODY CLEANSE (5-7 Days)

Upon Arising
Start this step on day two: Drink ¼ cup of fresh lemon or grapefruit juice mixed with 2 tablespoons olive oil and 3 oz. warm water.
Start of the Day
Drink 12 oz. Fresh apple juice diluted with 4 oz. Water; do this 3-4 times a day. Drink from morning to early afternoon.
In one of the apple juice drinks stir in 2 tablespoons of ground chia seed with 1 tablespoon Psyllium Husks. Mix thoroughly and drink.
2-7 p.m.
Drink vegetable juices between 1 p.m. To 7 p.m.
Vegetable juice recipe: 12 carrots, 1 head of celery, 4 apples, 1 head of spinach, 1 beet, 1 head parsley. Dilute the juice with 1/3 part water. If you feel full, do not force yourself to finish the batch. Save it for the next day.
Mix one of the veggie juice drinks with 1 tablespoons ground chia seed with 1 tablespoon Psyllium Husks
Bedtime
Combine ¼ cup freshly squeezed lemon or grapefruit juice with 2 tablespoons extra virgin olive oil. Drink without water and go to bed. Lay on your right side with your right knee to your chest for 20 minutes. This allows the oil to go directly to the gallbladder.

Cleanse The Body--Flush Away Toxins

Important reminder: Drink plenty of additional spring or purified water.

HOW TO BREAK THE FAST:

It is important to note that as you come off the cleanse the body has to re-adapt to eating solid foods. If you have too much solid food too fast, your stomach will be in pain and this can create more toxins in your body. So introduce foods slowly and use organic fruits and vegetables as much as possible. Follow the instructions below for the three days following the Mild Total Body Cleanse:

POST-CLEANSE DAY ONE:

Drink several 5-6 eight ounce glasses of freshly squeezed orange or grapefruit juice diluted with 5 oz. distilled water throughout the morning and mid-afternoon. For example, have a 12 oz. cup filled with 8 oz. of juice and 4 oz. of water. At this time you may have clear vegetable broth with ½ cup of steamed veggies.

POST-CLEANSE DAY TWO:

Drink fresh orange or grapefruit fruit juice all throughout the morning. By early afternoon drink 2-3 eight ounce glasses of carrot, apple, celery, and spinach juice diluted with 5 oz. of water. In the mid-afternoon enjoy one organic apple. In the evening have 1-2 cups lightly steamed vegetables for dinner with 1-2 cups of brown rice and a couple dashes of sea salt. Make sure to keep the meal simple without adding sauces.

POST-CLEANSE DAY THREE:

Drink orange or grapefruit juice in the morning followed by 2 cups raw (not dried) fruit and 2 tablespoons raw nuts for lunch. In the mid-afternoon have 1 eight ounce glass of carrot, apple, celery, and spinach juice diluted with 5 oz. of water. For dinner enjoy a veggie wrap with vegetables, sprouts, and hummus or olive oil on a sprouted grain tortilla.

3. EASY DOES IT LIVER CLEANSE

If you feel too restless to do the Total Body Cleanse start first with the mild cleanse. Once you have built up confidence you can do the Total Body Cleanse. You can follow up the mild cleanse with the Total Body Cleanse if you feel comfortable.

57

This cleanse is not a thorough cleanse but will begin to dissolve toxic liver bile and gallstones that have accumulated over time. Drink this elixir every morning 45 minutes before eating any other food for 10-20 days. During the day you can eat unlimited raw fruits (avoid dried fruit), vegetables (no potatoes), and 1-2 cups of brown rice. Avoid all other foods and make sure to drink around 64 oz. of purified drinking water.

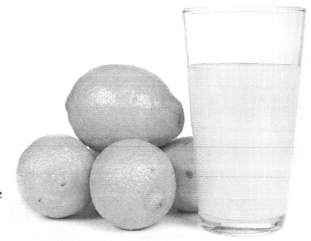

Ingredients:

½ cup warm purified water

2 tablespoons fresh lemon juice (raw)

1 tablespoon extra virgin olive oil

1 tablespoon black-strap molasses

1 pinch of cayenne pepper

Directions: Warm up water to body temperature and add all items, stir and drink.

4. ONE DAY GALLSTONE PURGE

The gallbladder supplies bile to the digestive tract that is mainly used to emulsify fats and oils and is a sack for holding some of the bile that the liver produces. In order to break down and digest fats, the liver must produce bile. When the liver is constantly stagnant, sediment often settles out of the bile and forms accumulations that resemble stones, sand or mud, in the gallbladder. Whether or not you have had your gallbladder removed, your liver is still producing bile in order to digest fats. The process of emulsification in the gallbladder and liver is best understood by the example of washing greasy dishes. It is nearly impossible to properly clean greasy dishes without soap as the soap emulsifies the fat so it can be removed. Similarly, the gallbladder stores bile and bile acids, which emulsify the fat you eat so it can be properly digested and transported through the intestine into the blood stream. This organ needs to be cleansed, otherwise bile can back up into the liver and cause major disruption in the filtering mechanism of the liver.

Here we have included the foods and herbs that cleanse the gallbladder.

Learn more about gallbladder health and solutions at www.gallbladderattack.com

NOTE: Those who have had their gallbladder removed cannot do this cleanse! If you have had your gallbladder removed you will want to take some form of bile salts (Beta Plus from Biotics Research, for example) with every meal for the rest of your life to prevent the good fats you eat from being flushed down the toilet. You should also be taking digestive enzymes with each meal to help break down the fats. Gallstone flushing has been used for centuries to purge the gallbladder from over-consumption of congesting foods.

THE GALLBLADDER CAN BE DAMAGED BY:

- Cold dairy products
- Excessive amounts of fat and oil
- Large amounts of spice
- Stress
- Very cold liquids

Symptoms of sediment in the gallbladder:

- Indigestion after eating any food or fatty or greasy foods
- Flatulence
- Periodic pain below the right side of the rib cage
- Tension in the back of the shoulder near the neck
- Bitter taste in the mouth and/or bitter fluid coming up after eating
- Chest pain
- Burping or belching
- Feeling of fullness or food not digesting
- Diarrhea (or alternating from soft to watery)
- Constipation
- Headache over eyes, especially on the right
- Frequent use of laxatives

THE GALLBLADDER IS PROTECTED BY:

NOTE: These foods do not have to be eaten alone in order to promote effectiveness; they can be eaten or juiced with other foods. Here are some foods and herbs and ideas on how to use them:

- **Apple cider vinegar**: Combine 2 oz. of apple cider vinegar, 8 oz. warm water, and 1 tablespoon raw honey. Drink first thing in the morning for 20 days.
- **Lemon juice and extra virgin olive oil**: Make a salad dressing with lemon juice, EVOO, and apple cider vinegar and drizzle over a salad of lettuce, radishes, apples, beets, and pumpkin seeds.
- **Radishes:** Eat raw or add them to a veggie juice (see juice recipes in **Chapter 7**).
- **Pears**: Eat raw, in salad or in juices.
- **Parsnips**: Add to salads, juices, and stir fries.
- **Lemons and limes:** Add to juices and soups, make homemade lemonade.
- **Seaweed:** Make seasoned brown rice with wakame seaweed and soy sauce.
- **Beets**: Grate up raw beet and put into a salad, or use in banana breads and juices. Or eat raw beets.

HERBS FOR GALLSTONE HEALTH:

NOTE: The best use of these herbs is to make herbal teas or take supplements that use some of these items.

- Gentian
- Dandelion
- Milk thistle
- Turmeric
- Celandine
- Peppermint oil
- Globe artichoke
- Fennel seed

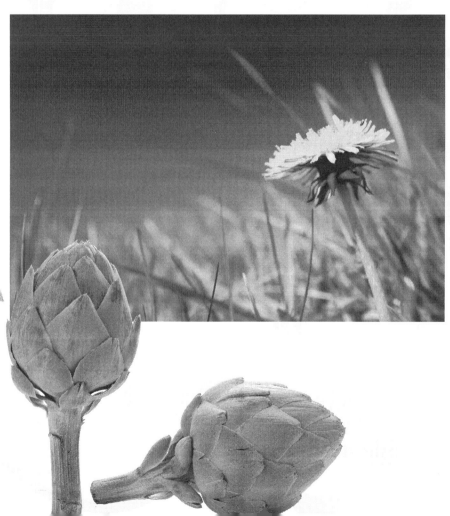

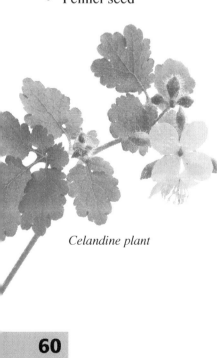

Celandine plant

INSTRUCTIONS:

Morning (8:00 a.m.-2:00 p.m.):
Juice 12 apples and dilute with 1/3 part water. Drink this mixture throughout the morning to early mid-afternoon.

Mid-afternoon (2:00-7:00 p.m.):
Throughout the afternoon from 2-7 p.m., drink a total of 25 oz. of vegetable juice - 10 carrots, 2 apples, 10 radishes, 2 pears, 1 lemon, 1 beet, and 1 head parsley.
Dilute the juice with 1/3 part water.
If you feel full, do not force yourself to finish the batch.

Bedtime:
Combine 2/3 cup extra virgin olive oil, slightly warmed, with 2/3 cup freshly squeezed lemon or grapefruit juice. Stir together, drink, stir, and drink until you have finished the mixture. Without drinking any water, go directly to bed and lay on your right side with your right knee to your chest for 20 minutes. This allows the oil to go directly to the gallbladder.

CONCLUSION:

Congratulations! You have accomplished a thorough cleanse of your body from top to bottom! You are what we call a new creation. Now that you are done with one of the above cleanses, be cautious about the foods you choose to put into your body. You've cleared out thousands of toxins accumulated over many years in your body. It is wise to use the rest of the Food Beautiful Principles to create a temperate diet that will increase the quality of your life. Use your willpower and good judgment to select and eat life-giving foods in proper combinations, regardless of the ridicule of friends and family. Rest assured you are doing the utmost to ensure your own good health.

Consume Healing Foods--Avoid Deceptive Foods

- Top Reasons to Eat Organic
- What Grandma Used to Know--Healing Properties of Foods
- Remedies and Guidelines for Your Disease

Nearly 2,500 years ago Hippocrates is purported to have said, "Let food be thy medicine, and medicine be thy food." Hippocrates was indeed onto something good, that the food we choose to eat can prevent and in some cases fight disease. God created all plant-based foods with an abundance of living enzymes and nutrients encoded within them to heal and restore the body. Natural, unprocessed plant-based foods have specific uses that prevent and even restore health. When you eat cooked and processed foods, your body is robbed of living enzymes, minerals, vitamins, and co-factors needed to create new healthy living cells. Dead foods may satisfy your hunger for a time, but at a great cost to your health. A healthy cell will reproduce a healthy cell and a sick cell will reproduce a sick cell. The integrity of a cell's health is based upon what you feed it. If you feel sick and tired, you will stay sick and tired unless you change what you are currently doing. Instead, make better choices by choosing living foods replete with vital nutrients which will automatically restore energy and healing to repair degenerative tissue.

Every plant-based food that grows from the earth produces a specific biological action that manifests health and strength within you. When specific foods like ginger and garlic are added to the diet, your body boosts its natural immune system function while reducing cholesterol, stress, pain, inflammation, allergies, osteoarthritis, and

> "He who does not know food, how can he understand the diseases of man?"
> - *Hippocrates, the father of medicine (460-357 B.C.)*

> "People are applying the precautionary principle to their own lives by purchasing food that has not been produced by industrial methods, from the simple stance of hazard avoidance. Organically produced food is the best option that we have."
> - *Dr. Vyvyan Howard, toxico-pathologist at the University of Liverpool, UK*

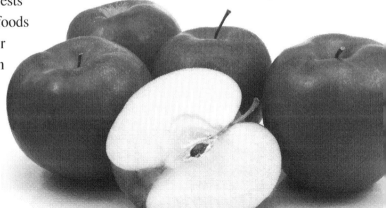

much more. In this chapter, I address the top ten reasons why plant-based organic foods are the healing solution for a sick body and an even sicker environment. In this chapter you will also find which foods and herbs can help you overcome both disease and pain.

It is time to embrace change, with an open mind and willingness to make your body and earth healthier, so future generations can thrive and the life-enhancing habits we adopt can sustain life. Start healing yourself today from seasonal allergies, asthma, sinusitis, hay fever, and other illnesses by consuming healing herbs and foods.

"The burden of food-related ill health measured in terms of mortality and morbidity is similar to that attributable to smoking... The vast majority of the burden is attributable to unhealthy diets rather than to food-borne diseases."
- *Journal of Epidemiology and Community Health*

TOP REASONS TO BUY ORGANIC

Organic food contributes to a healthy body in many ways. Here are the top ten reasons to buy and eat organic. Eating organic food:

1. KEEPS TOXIC CHEMICALS OUT OF YOUR BODY.

Non-organic fruits and vegetables are treated with pesticides, herbicides, and fungicides, which are all poisons designed to kill living organisms and can be harmful to humans. Many pesticides were registered and approved for use by the EPA long before any research was conducted that linked these chemicals to cancer and other diseases. The Organic Trade Association (OTA) concluded that 60% of all herbicides, 90% of all fungicides and 30% of all insecticides are cancer-causing. In addition to cancer, these pesticides are linked to birth defects, nerve damage, genetic mutations, vitamin and mineral deficiency, accelerated aging and hormonal imbalances. According to the National Academy of Science, "Neurological and behavioral effects may result from low-level exposure to pesticides." The following is a report from the Environmental Working Group (EWG), a nonprofit consumer advocate group comprised of scientists, lawyers, policy experts, engineers and computer programmers committed to exposing threats to our health and the environment. EWG put together the "Shopper's Guide to Pesticide in Produce," ranking the pesticide contamination of 47 popular fruits and vegetables. Those below a combined score of 40 are considered safe. This report does not indicate the depletion of nutritional value from using fertilizers and pesticides.

Pesticide Rank and Contamination Combined Score of 47 Fruits and Vegetables:

Rank	Food	Score		Rank	Food	Score
1	Peaches	100		26	Mushrooms	36
2	Strawberries	89		27	Cantaloupe	36
3	Apples	88		28	Sweet potatoes	35
4	Spinach	85		29	Grapefruit	34
5	Nectarines	85		30	Winter squash	34
6	Celery	83		31	Blueberries	30
7	Pears	80		32	Watermelon	27
8	Cherries	76		33	Plums	26
9	Potatoes	67		34	Tangerines	25
10	Sweet bell pepper	66		35	Cabbage	25
11	Raspberries	66		36	Papaya	23
12	Grapes, imported	64		37	Kiwi	23
13	Carrots	57		38	Bananas	19
14	Green beans	57		39	Broccoli	18
15	Hot peppers	55		40	Onions	17
16	Oranges	53		41	Asparagus	16
17	Apricots	51		42	Sweet peas	13
18	Cucumber	51		43	Mango	12
19	Tomatoes	48		44	Cauliflower	10
20	Collard greens	48		45	Pineapples	6
21	Grapes, domestic	47		46	Avocado	4
22	Turnip greens	41		47	Sweet corn	1
23	Honeydew melons	40				
24	Lettuce	40				
25	Kale	39				

The National Cancer Institute found that farmers exposed to herbicides had a six times greater risk of contracting cancer than non-agricultural workers. In California, pesticide poisonings among farm workers have risen an average of 14% per year since 1973. Field workers suffer the highest risk of occupational illnesses in the state of Colorado. Stay safe and buy organic.

2. TASTES BETTER AND HAS MORE NUTRITIVE CONTENT THAN NON-ORGANIC FOODS.

One of the best methods for removing all toxins, pesticides, viruses, and mold from produce is to soak it in water with two tablespoons of raw apple cider vinegar for 15 minutes. Then using gloves, remove from water and rinse under purified water.

Researchers have found that most organic foods taste better and have more vitamins, minerals, and phytonutrients gram for gram than conventionally farmed produce! Conventional farmers add phosphorus, nitrogen and potassium to the soil. They rarely, if ever, add essential minerals back into the soil. In conventional farming, when a field is not allowed to lie fallow every few years, the mineral content in soil is depleted, causing a substantial decline in the nutritional value of food. Additionally, conventional farming uses chemicals that kill beneficial bacteria which enhance the plant's ability to synthesize and absorb nutrients. Organic farming practices increase the number of beneficial soil organisms resulting in more nutritious and tasty vegetation. Most organic farmers use highly nutritive compost like kelp meal, alpaca manure, and sustainable compost which contain dozens of different trace minerals and soil builders. Many organic farmers practice crop rotation so that other plants replenish nutrients used up during the previous growing season. This practice preserves the soil's nutrient composition so it can be used again the following season.

Most small farmers have been displaced by the huge agri-businesses (large farms) that receive almost all the governmental subsidies as well as most of the profits. Agri-business funnels millions of dollars into the pockets of politicians every election. The government only gives lip service to healthy foods; frankly, there is no profit or political payoff growing organic foods. Do yourself and local organic farmers a favor and make a choice to buy locally grown organic foods!

TIP: Buy in bulk when organic apples, carrots, and beets are on sale, and then in the fall store them in a cool dry basement inside a container filled with sand. The foods will last all winter long.

3. HELPS YOU AVOID GMO FOODS.

GMO stands for "Genetically Modified Organism." A GMO plant is created when a foreign gene replaces the original gene. The gene comes from a variety of sources (animal, plant, bacteria, etc...) and is inserted into the plant to increase its color, growth, and appearance. Biotechnology corporations argue that their genetic manipulations are similar to the plant's natural evolution or to traditional reproduction techniques. This is false. Crossing different species does not occur in nature. Even if the gene itself is not dangerous or toxic, it could alter complex biochemical systems that create new bioactive compounds, or change the concentrations of those that are normally present. Gene manipulation can and has already introduced new toxins, illnesses, allergies, and weaknesses in humans and animals. GMO's can cause side effects that cannot be anticipated or controlled.

One big GMO food to avoid is canola oil. It was developed through the hybridization of rape seed and lear. Rape seed oil is toxic because it contains significant amounts of a poisonous substance called erucic acid. Engineered as a super oil with no need to be sprayed with pesticides, it is so toxic that bugs will not touch it. America's large agri-com businesses can market it as organic, because it requires no pesticides. Rapeseed was never given GRAS (Generally Recognized as Safe) status by the U.S. Food and Drug Administration, so a change in regulation was needed before canola oil could be marketed in the U.S. Somehow GRAS status was granted in 1985, for which, it is rumored, the Canadian government spent $50 million. Read more in MG Enig and SW Fallon's "The Oiling of America" and in the Canola Oil Cover Up at **www.westonaprice. org/knowyourfats/canola.html**.

With conventional farming, the soil is used more as a medium for holding plants in a vertical position so they can be chemically fertilized, resulting in 40-50% fewer nutrients compared to organic vegetable gardening which results in 50% more vitamins, minerals, enzymes, and phytonutrients.

GMO foods:
- Damage the ecosystem, harming wild life and natural habitats.
- Transfer their genetic modifications to natural organisms, making the new organism unable to return to its original state.
- Increase pollution in food and water supplies because GMO's have an increased resistance to bacteria that results in the need to triple the amount of herbicides used on crops.
- Cause unpredictable and permanent changes in the action and nature of our food; a new GMO can give rise to novel proteins in our food with unknown results for our health.

- Reduce beneficial properties in foods.
- Reduce effectiveness of antibiotics in humans.
- Cause allergic reactions in humans.
- Can cause permanent damage to human DNA, thus creating a host of new diseases in our body and in future generations.
- Suppress the human immune system and increase our susceptibility to illness and disease.
- Cause livestock to become infected with various bacteria such as E. coli.

Unless these foods are certified organic they are a Genetically Modified Organism: Soy, Wheat, Corn, Tomatoes, Peppers, and Peanuts. Check out What foods to Avoid In the **Appendix 1** and **2**

4. REDUCES CONTAMINANTS IN WATER!

Water makes up 75% of the human body mass and covers 75% of the planet. Despite the fact that water is integral to life, the Environmental Protection Agency (EPA) estimates that pesticides – most of which are cancer-causing – now contaminate the groundwater in 38 states and pollute the primary source of drinking water for more than half the country's population, resulting in more diseases and illnesses than ever recorded. Other emerging issues are the prescription drugs and hormones being leached into the water supply through groundwater and sewage plants. The hormone molecule is too small to be completely filtered out in most water purification systems, but can be greatly reduced.

If you buy and eat organic foods, you are supporting farmers who do not pollute our groundwater with pesticides and other chemicals.

5. HELPS YOU AVOID BACTERIA.

The 21st century started out as the age of dangerous food contamination. Over the last few years, we have been bombarded with news stories reporting the outbreak of E. coli in spinach and salmonella in tomatoes and lemons. In June of 2008, the FDA released statements informing the public about a salmonella outbreak, which they initially believed could be traced back to tomatoes. Later, they changed their story and claimed that the source was jalapeno peppers. When the researchers attempt to determine the root cause in any of these cases, the trail always leads back to the true culprit, the fecal matter of livestock. Our hooved animals and chickens are confined in large numbers and fed recycled animal parts and grains contaminated with pesticides and genetically modified proteins. As a result, disease-causing bacteria is shed in their excrement which is then used as fertilizer. Due to worldwide food safety issues and the inconsistency from country to country of food purity standards, growing your own fruit and vegetables or buying locally grown organic food ensures healthy, nutritious meals for you and your family.

6. SAVES ENERGY AND HELPS US "GO GREEN".

American farms have changed drastically in the last three generations, from family-based small businesses dependent on human energy to large-scale factory farms dependent on fossil fuels. Modern farming uses more petroleum than any other single industry, consuming 12 percent of the country's total energy supply. More energy is now used to produce fertilizers than to till, cultivate, and harvest all the crops in the United States. Organic farming is still mainly based on labor-intensive practices such as weeding by hand and using green manures and crop covers rather than synthetic fertilizers to build up soil. You will help save money and energy while producing less waste when you support your local organic food sources. The food is picked fresh ensuring the best nutritional value and taste.

TIPS:
- Help lessen the impact of waste products in city dumps by composting leftover food.
- When gardening, help lessen green waste by composting and mulching.
- Help lessen air pollution created from conventional lawn yard-care equipment.
- Provide a diverse species of plants to serve as a habitat for beneficial insects and wildlife.

7. SUPPORTS LOCAL FARMERS AND YOUR LOCAL ECONOMY.

Most organic farms are small, independently-owned and operated family farms of less than 100 acres, although some large farms are converting to organic practices. It is estimated that the United States has lost more than 655,000 family farms in the past decade. Although organic foods are more expensive than conventional foods, conventional food prices do not reflect the hidden costs which burden taxpayers, including nearly $92 billion in federal subsidies in 2004. Other hidden costs include pesticide regulation and testing, hazardous waste disposal, clean-up and environmental damage. Dr. Gary Null, author of "The Complete Guide to Health and Nutrition says, "If you add in the real environmental and social costs of irrigation to a head of lettuce, its price can range between $2 and $3." An abundance of studies proves that most of the money spent supporting local farmers stays within your local community; whereas, very little of the money spent in big box food stores, both chains and franchises, remains in your town.

8. IS SO EASY YOU CAN GROW YOUR OWN.

Plant a plot in a community garden, a garden in your back yard, a container garden on your apartment patio, or a hydroponics vegetable garden in your house. There is no fresher, more nutritious, or cost-effective way to stock your house with organic foods than growing them yourself. When you take control over your own food through organic gardening, you avoid the loss of enzymes and nutrients through irradiation, synthetic fertilizers, and chemical pesticides. Also, you do not pay the "middle man" in addition to rising shipping costs due to escalating fuel prices and road taxes.

Organic farming provides:

1. Reduced food costs.
2. Reduced mystery diseases and chronic immunological and hormone related diseases.
3. Abundant fresh food that has not been grown with pesticides and chemical fertilizers.
4. An education for our children in ecology, botany, and the cycle of life.
5. A fun and healthy family activity that encourages exercise.

9. ENSURES A SUSTAINABLE FUTURE FOR OUR CHILDREN.

Supporting organic farming benefits your family and everyone's families by reducing toxic pollutants in the air, water, soil, and our bodies. According to the August 2002 issue of Science Magazine, the drift of synthetic fertilizers emitted by industrial farms has caused a dead zone in the delicate ecosystem of the Gulf of Mexico larger than the State of New Jersey. If this goes unchecked, our children will not have a world to live in.

For every $100 dollars spent in local stores, $43 dollars stays in the community. Of every $100 spent in big box stores, only $11 stays in the community.

During World War II, American families planted "patriotic gardens" in an effort to support our troops, while at the same time providing optimally nutritious foods for their families.

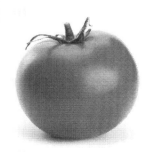

WHAT GRANDMA USED TO KNOW--HEALING PROPERTIES OF FOODS

Food is so common in our daily routine that we tend to overlook the potential wealth of health inside of it. As our grandmothers knew when they fed us our fruit and veggies, you can beat some of the toughest diseases out there by simply incorporating the right foods into your diet.

The body is continually producing new cells. In order for these cells to be healthy and full of life, they need to have the right foundation, nutrients, and energy. In the same way, life for a plant requires soil (organic food), water, and sunlight (energy). If you watered a plant with only soda, for example, instead of water, it would eventually die. Dead food cannot bring life to a plant or a human. Only life can beget life.

If you get sick frequently or have a disease, examine the foods you are eating. Are they dead foods? When dead foods enter the body they lack both the right enzymes and nutrients to sustain life for long.

The best thing we can do for our body is feed it the food our Creator designed for it. The list below provides the healing properties of several varieties of food:

HEALING PROPERTIES OF FRUIT

AMALAKI is widely considered the most rejuvenating super fruit. It promotes healthy eyes and strengthens the liver. It promotes healthy brain function and fortifies the heart. It also helps to maintain normal blood sugar levels and reduces acidity in the body. It is anti-inflammatory and strengthens the nervous system and enhances memory function.

APPLES help moisten dryness in the lungs, protect the lungs from cigarette smoke, have a beneficial effect on low blood sugar conditions, and stimulate appetite. Apples help the body overcome indigestion, due in part to the presence of malic and tartic acids, which inhibit the growth of fermented food and disease-producing bacteria in the digestive tract. They also contain pectin, which removes cholesterol, toxic metals (such as lead and mercury), and radiation contamination. Apples and their juice are cleansing for the liver and gallbladder and help to soften gallstones.

APRICOTS helps to moisten lung conditions such as asthma, bronchitis, and pneumonia. Due to their high copper and cobalt content, apricots are commonly suggested for those suffering from anemia and constipation.

AVOCADOS helps build up red blood cells, calm liver conditions, and lubricate the lungs and intestines. Avocados are a natural source of lecithin, a brain food, and more than 80% of their calories come from easily digested, primarily polyunsaturated fat. They are rich in copper and potassium, which aid in red blood cell formation. Avocados are also a great protein source, often recommended for nursing mothers, athletes, children, and the elderly.

BANANAS helps the body overcome constipation and ulcers if eaten when ripe. Bananas eaten before they are completely ripened will halt diarrhea, colitis, and hemorrhoids. They also help to cleanse drugs from the body, which is useful for those trying to overcome drug addictions (especially alcoholism). They are rich in potassium and easy to digest; bananas aid those with hypertension and high blood pressure.

BLACKBERRIES are similar in effect to raspberries (see raspberries).

CANTELOUPE helps to clean out the liver by stimulating bile flow (when eaten on an empty stomach). The seeds also contain healing properties that are helpful to overcome depression. Make sure to eat the seeds while eating the fruit and save the ones you can't eat for a later snack.

CHERRIES are a well-known remedy for gout, arthritis, and rheumatism, and help overcome numbness in the limbs and paralysis as a result of rheumatism. Their rich iron content makes them useful for treating anemia.

FIGS are one of nature's most alkalinizing foods, perfect for those who eat highly refined foods and meats, which are acidic. Figs help with dysentery and hemorrhoids, act as a detoxifier in the colon, cleanse the intestines and help iron absorption. They can be used to clear up skin boils and discharge, and are high in mucin, which has a soothing laxative affect.

GOJI BERRIES are from the Himalayas near Tibet. They are a rich source of Vitamin C, with 500 times more per ounce than oranges. They are also a superb source of Vitamin A, with more beta-carotene than carrots. They contain other vitamins such as B1, B2, B6, and E. They are also a rich source of both selenium and germanium, have 18 amino acids (higher than bee pollen) and 21 trace minerals, linoleic acid, and other beneficial food co-factors. Goji berries strengthen the immune system and may help to stimulate the release of human growth hormone by the pituitary gland.

GRAPES have tannins in the dark varieties that act as natural antioxidants. They also contain carotenoids, which prevent the oxidation of fats that leads to hardening of the arteries. Grapes build and purify the blood and improve the cleansing function of the glands. This benefits the liver and kidneys and thus strengthens their corresponding tissues: the bones and sinews. Grapes provide positive affects for those with arthritis, rheumatism, edema, and urinary difficulty. To overcome anemia, combine raisins with raw honey and consume twice a day. For relieving a dry cough, consume a concoction of grapes with honey twice a day.

GRAPEFRUIT helps with poor digestion, belching, increases in appetite during pregnancy, alcohol intoxication, allergies, hay fever, strep throat, Candida overgrowth, giardia, athlete's foot, parasites, flu, staph infections, nail fungi, dandruff, yeast infections, sinus problems, and ear infections. Eating the grapefruit peel regulates digestive energy, resolves mucus conditions of the lungs, and can treat lung congestion and coughs. The bioflavonoid and Vitamin C in the fruit and its peel strengthens the gums, the arteries, and circulation in general. To extract properties from the peel, place it fresh into simmering water for 20 minutes, strain the liquid and drink the tea.

LEMONS & LIMES are natural astringents, antiseptics, and antimicrobials. They help with weight loss, blood cleansing, high blood pressure, poor circulation, and weak blood vessels. Lemons and limes destroy putrefactive bacteria in the intestines and mouth, and are mucus-resolving for dysentery, colds, flu, hacking cough, and parasite infestation. They benefit the action of the liver by encouraging the formation of bile, which improves the absorption of minerals.

MANGO is high in iron, so pregnant women and people with anemia are advised to eat this fruit regularly. Mango is a rich source of Vitamin A (beta-carotene), E, and selenium, which help to protect against heart disease and other ailments. Mango also helps to combat acidity, poor digestion, constipation, respiratory problems, fever, and kidney problems including nephritis. Eat mangos while traveling in other countries as the healing properties in the fruit kill giardia and other parasites.

MULBERRY helps to build blood, moisten the lungs and gastrointestinal tract, and strengthen the liver and kidneys. Mulberry is used to treat vertigo, paralysis, stomach ulcers, diabetes, dry cough, ringing in the ears, and poor joint mobility. It is also beneficial for blood deficiencies (such as anemia), prematurely graying hair, irritability, insomnia, and constipation caused by lack of fluids.

ORANGE provides a general tonic for weak digestion, poor appetite, inflammation, high acidic diseases, arthritis, and high fevers. The peel has stimulating, digestive, and mucus-resolving properties similar to the grapefruit peel.

PAPAYA strengthens the stomach, acts as a digestive aid, alleviates coughing, is used for dysentery, indigestion, excess mucus, and pain from rheumatism. Under-ripe papaya has a high amount of papain, an enzyme good for digesting protein and breaking down deposits on the teeth. Papaya has a vermicidal action capable of destroying most intestinal worms and also contains carpain, an anti-tumor activity compound.

PEACHES help moisten the lungs, are used for dry cough, and help to lower high blood pressure. Peaches are a natural astringent and tend to limit perspiration while tightening tissues (when used in topical creams). The kernel inside the peach seed strengthens blood circulation, is used in anti-tumor formulas and for those with uterine fibroids. Peach leaf taken as a tea destroys worms.

PEARS are a great fruit for balancing blood sugar in people with diabetes. The pear also helps to strengthen the voice and clear up coughing, gallbladder inflammation, and obstructions.

PERSIMMON is used to moisten the lungs, reduce phlegm, soothe the mucus lining of the digestive tract, and halt gastrointestinal inflammations, canker sores, and chronic bronchitis. Unripe persimmons have high amounts of tannic acid, which is helpful for treating diarrhea, dysentery, vomiting blood, and coughing up mucus.

PINEAPPLES quench thirst by supplying electrolytes and minerals to the body. Pineapples help individuals overcome sunstroke, indigestion, anorexia, diarrhea, and edema. They contain an enzyme called bromelain that increases digestive ability, acts as an anti-inflammatory, and destroys worms in the colon/intestines. Ripe pineapples contain large amounts of bromelain which is most beneficial for those with severe disc inflammations. Note: those with peptic ulcers or skin discharges should not use pineapple.

PLUMS are used for liver disease and diabetes, cirrhosis of the liver, hardened or expanded liver conditions, dehydration, and poor assimilation of carbohydrates. The Umeboshi salt plum treats indigestion and diarrhea, removes worms, and stops dysentery.

POMEGRANATE helps to destroy worms in the intestinal tract, strengthens gums, and soothes ulcers of the mouth and throat. It is also loaded with Vitamin C and iron, which is helpful for strengthening low immune systems and addressing anemia.

RASPBERRIES enrich and cleanse the blood of toxins, regulate the menstrual cycle, and control urinary function and anemia as well as excessive urination (especially at night). The raspberry leaf strengthens the uterus, balances excessive menstrual flow, and restrains bleeding in general.

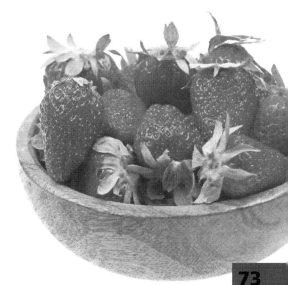

STRAWBERRIES improve appetite, moisten the lungs, and are used for thirst, sore throat, and hoarseness. Eating strawberries before meals helps combat poor digestion which is accompanied by abdominal pain and swelling.

Strawberries also help to relieve urinary difficulties, painful urination and inability to urinate. Rich in silicon and Vitamin C, they are also useful for arterial and all connective tissue repairs. As they are one of the first fruits to appear in spring, they are helpful for cleansing the body. Those who are allergic to strawberries, for the most part, are those who eat the unripened and non-organic fruit.

WATERMELON is cooling and great for quenching thirst in the summer and supplying electrolytes after a workout. Watermelon aids those with urinary difficulty, edema (water retention), canker sores, depression, and kidney and urinary tract inflammations. The seed of the watermelon contains cucurbocitrin, a nutrient that dilates capillaries, lowering cholesterol. The rind is useful for high blood pressure, diabetes, and calcium needs. Watermelon rind and seeds can be juiced.

HEALING PROPERTIES OF LEGUMES

ADUKI BEAN aids the adrenals and kidneys, detoxifies the body, reduces swelling in the lower body, and acts as a natural diuretic. Beneficial for conditions such as jaundice, diarrhea, edema, and boils, the aduki bean also promotes weight loss. If you experience prolonged menstruation, chew five raw aduki beans thoroughly daily until menses stops.

BLACK BEAN benefits kidneys and reproductive functions and is used to help relieve low back pain, knee pain, infertility, and involuntary seminal emission.

BLACK SOYBEAN improves blood circulation and water metabolism, acts as a diuretic, removes toxins from the body and is used to treat rheumatism and kidney disease.

CAROB is a safe alternative to the cocoa bean with twice the amount of calcium, half the amount of fat, and no phenylethylamins (a molecule that can trigger migraines). Carob is high in proteins, rich in pectin fiber, and no sweetener is needed to enhance its flavor. In addition, carob helps treat diarrhea (especially in infants), inactivate toxins and bacteria growth.

FAVA BEAN strengthens the spleen and pancreas and is used as a diuretic to treat edema and swelling.

GARBANZO BEAN is beneficial to the pancreas, stomach, and heart and helps balance blood sugar in diabetics.

KIDNEY BEAN is a natural diuretic that can be used in treating edema and swelling. For hundreds of years the ripe bean pod has been used to heal kidney and bladder pain. This then helped individuals overcome rheumatism and chronic edema (water retention).

LENTIL is beneficial to the heart and circulation and stimulates the adrenal system.

LIMA BEAN is highly alkalinizing and benefits the lung and liver. The bean neutralizes acidic conditions such as those that arise from excessive meat and refined food consumption.

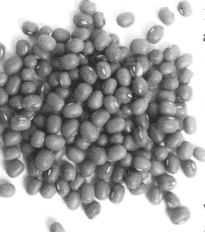

MUNG BEAN detoxifies the body, benefits the liver and gallbladder, acts as a diuretic, and reduces swelling in the lower legs. Mung bean is used as a cure for food poisoning (drink liquid from mung soup), dysentery (cook with garlic), diarrhea, painful urination, mumps, burns, lead and pesticide poisoning, boils, heat stroke, conjunctivitis, and edema (especially in the lower extremities). It is also beneficial for treating high blood pressure, acidosis, gastro-intestinal ulcers, skin outbreaks, thirst, and restlessness.

PEA helps to harmonize digestion and reduces the effects of an overworked, jam-packed liver so digestion in the stomach as well as pancreas and spleen function will improve. Peas also reduce vomiting, belching, hiccups and coughing and are mildly laxative. Peas are also used for spasms, edema, constipation, and skin eruptions such as carbuncles and boils.

SOYBEAN, when used occasionally in small amounts, improves almost all organs, cleanses blood vessels and heart by improving circulation, promotes clear vision, acts as a diuretic, lowers fever, eliminates toxins from the body, boosts milk secretion in nursing mothers, and acts as a remedy for dizziness. It is also good for toxemia during pregnancy, food poisoning, and is a natural source of lecithin (good food for the brain). Young children usually easily digest soybeans when they are steamed or fermented. However, overcooked soybeans can inhibit the digestive enzyme, trypsin, making them hard to digest. It is best to use the fermented types of soy: tempeh, tofu, and miso. If used too much, soybeans can cause anemia, amenorrhea, osteoporosis, weakened kidney and adrenal function, hypothyroidism, and mineral deficiencies.

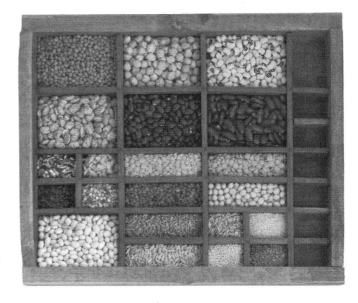

STRING BEAN is used to balance diabetes, frequent urination, and thirst.

Herbal Combinations For Better Digestion and Taste of Legumes

Legume	Suggested Herb Combination
Garbanzo, Lentil	Mint, Garlic
Lentil, Mung, Black, Aduki	Coriander, Cumin, Ginger
Lentil, Garbanzo, Split Pea	Dill, Basil
Black Pinto, Lentil, Kidney	Sage, Thyme, Oregano
Pinto, Kidney	Fennel, Cumin, Garlic, Onion
All	Add seaweeds (Kombu or Kelp) to legumes while cooking to make them more digestible and tastier.

HEALING PROPERTIES OF GRAINS

AMARANTH is used to help fulfill protein and calcium requirements. It benefits the lungs, and is high in protein, fiber, amino acids, Vitamin C, and calcium.

BARLEY has a cooling nature that strengthens the spleen and pancreas, regulates the stomach, builds blood (for the elderly, children, and anemic persons), and benefits the gallbladder and nerves. It is also easily digested, alleviates painful and difficult urination, quells fever, and helps reduce tumors, swelling, and edema. This grain can be more difficult to digest for those dealing with Celiac Disease.

BROWN RICE soothes the stomach, expels toxins, balances blood sugar, and is hypoallergenic (safe for those with wheat allergies and Candida). Since it has a concentration of B Vitamins, it is highly beneficial for calming the nerves and relieving mental tension and depression. A handful of raw brown rice thoroughly chewed, as the only food in the morning, helps to expel worms.

BUCKWHEAT cleanses and strengthens intestines and improves appetite. It is helpful for dysentery and chronic diarrhea, strengthens capillaries and blood vessels, reduces blood pressure, and increases circulation to the hands and feet. Buckwheat is actually a seed, not a grain, and is not a member of the wheat family. It is extremely dense in protein and B Vitamins.

CORN helps to improve the appetite, regulate digestion, and strengthen the kidneys. Corn silk is a fast and effective diuretic and can be used as a tea infusion for urinary difficulty, high blood pressure, edema, kidney stones, and gallstones.

KAMUT, called the "Ancient Wheat," is great for those sensitive to today's wheat and other glutinous products. Kamut is high in protein and other nutrients.

MILLET is a natural diuretic, which also strengthens kidneys while benefiting digestion. It is highly alkalinizing, sweetens the breath by retarding bacterial growth, helps prevent miscarriage and is an antifungal (best grain for those with Candida). Millet is useful for diarrhea (roast millet before cooking), indigestion, diabetes, and to soothe morning sickness (eat millet soup).

OATS help to restore the nervous and reproductive systems and remove cholesterol from the digestive tract and arteries. It is rich in silicon, which helps renew the bones and connective tissue. Oats are also nourishing for young children to help their bodies develop the nervous system. Cooked oatmeal (cooled) has been used to sooth burns on the skin. Make a paste with water and oats and apply to the affected area, allowing it to sit for 15-20 minutes.

QUINOA is extremely high in protein, iron, B Vitamins, Vitamin E, and has more calcium than milk. It also helps to strengthen the kidneys and the pericardium functions.

RYE increases endurance, aids muscle formation, cleanses and renews arteries, and aids fingernail, hair and bone formation. It is high in complex low glycemic carbohydrates, potassium, and B Vitamins.

red quinoa

SPELT strengthens the spleen and pancreas functions, and especially benefits the frail and deficient person. Spelt is often used for treating diarrhea, constipation, poor digestion, colitis, and other intestinal disorders.

WHEAT has been known to encourage growth, weight gain, and fat formation, which is good for children and frail people. It should be eaten in small amounts, if at all, by obese individuals and those with growths or tumors. Wheat can provoke allergic reactions as the flour becomes rancid from oxidation within two weeks after grinding. Wheat flour should be used right after grinding; otherwise, it needs to be kept in an airtight container, refrigerated, and used within two weeks.

HEALING PROPERTIES OF NUTS AND SEEDS

The best way to eat seeds or nuts is to soak them overnight in water to initiate their sprouting process. This makes the protein and fats more digestible. Drain the water and dry them, then eat them raw or lightly roasted. Store hulled seeds in dark glass bottles in cold places. Do not store in plastic, as the oil-rich food combines with the plastic to form plasticides.

ALMONDS help to relieve stagnant mucus in the lungs, alleviate coughs, and lubricate the intestines. They are also used for lung conditions including coughing and asthma. The almond is the only nut to alkalinize the blood. Almonds help to raise hemoglobin, form new blood cells, and enable liver, heart, brain and nerves to perform their respective functions normally. The nut prolongs life, and tones and energizes muscle function and brain power. To help relieve lung conditions, make the raw almond milk recipe found at the back of this book. You can purchase organic raw almonds online at www.realrawfood.com. To relieve asthma, bronchitis, and whooping cough, mix 10-15 drops each of ginger and lemon juices to a spoonful of almond oil and take for 10-15 days at a stretch once or twice a day. For healthy skin, mix equal parts rose petal paste, almond paste (from blanched almonds), and milk cream. Apply twice daily over face, and it will beautify the face, moisturizing and nourishing the skin, removing black-heads and pimples, retarding the effects of premature aging on the face, and bringing back that healthy glow and softness to your skin.

BRAZIL NUT has a large amount of selenium and chromium, indeed its selenium content is in higher concentrations than any other food. Selenium is a major antioxidant that protects the cell membrane from degeneration and decreases the risk of cancer and heart disease. Medical surveys show a direct correlation between high amounts of selenium and decreased risk of colon, breast, lung and prostate cancer. Selenium also preserves tissue elasticity, and reduces allergies and inflammation. Selenium also helps in the prevention and treatment of dandruff.

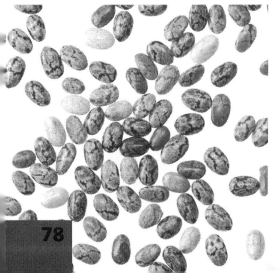

CHIA SEED has been used by South American and Aztec communities for thousands of centuries as a high energy endurance food that is still called the "running food." This seed is the highest source of Omega-3 fatty acids – more than flax seed! Chia seeds offer a disease-fighting arsenal of antioxidants, including chlorogenic acid, caffeic acid, myricetin, quercetin and flavonols. Chia seeds are used to help people overcome mineral, vitamin, and protein deficiencies. It is also helpful for those with diabetes, high blood pressure, hypoglycemia and high cholesterol.

CITRUS SEED EXTRACT is extremely beneficial as it is a natural antibiotic, antifungal, and anti-bacterial. It inhibits many types of microbes such as parasites (protozoa, amoebas, bacteria, viruses) and 30 types of fungus, including Candida yeast-like fungi.

COCONUT is used for strengthening the overall body, eliminating fungal infections, killing adult amoebas inside the body, emaciation, nosebleeds, and childhood malnutrition. Coconut milk is helpful in treating edema resulting from heart weakness and diabetes. There are also many claims that coconut oil helps those with an under-active thyroid.

FLAX SEED is a natural and mild laxative, relieves pain and in-flammation, is a rich source of Omega-3 fatty acids, and pulls out excess estrogen in the blood. The seed helps increase cognitive function and balance hormones in the body. It also helps to alleviate constipation, high blood pressure, poor eye site, depression, arthritis, and allergies.

PEANUTS should be used with caution! Buy only organic as peanuts have a carcinogenic fungus that grows inside the nut and are heavily sprayed with chemicals and synthetic fertilizers. They should be avoided by those who are overweight and those who have cancer or yeast infections. Peanuts are used to increase the milk supply of nursing mothers, stop bleeding, including hemophilia and blood in the urine, and help to lower blood pressure (drink tea of peanut shells).

PINE NUT is mildly laxative, helpful for dizziness, dry cough, spitting up blood, and constipation.

PISTACHIO influences proper function of the liver and the kidney, purifies the blood, lubricates the intestines, and is beneficial for constipation. It is an important tonic for the whole body when eaten raw.

PUMPKIN & SQUASH SEEDS influence optimal function of the colon and spleen-pancreas. They are a diuretic and a vermifuge (expel worms such as tape worms and round worms). These seeds are also beneficial for those with motion sickness, nausea, impotency, and swollen prostate. They are a great source of zinc and Omega-3 fatty acids.

SESAME SEED (BLACK) helps strengthen the liver and kidneys, lubricate the intestines, strength-en the heart, spleen-pancreas, and lungs. It is also used to relieve rheumatism, constipation, dry cough, blurry vision, ringing in ears, blood in urine, low back pain, weak knees, stiff joints, nervous spasm, dandruff, headaches, insufficient mother's milk, dizziness, and numbness.

SUNFLOWER SEED influences optimal function of the spleen-pancreas, acts as an energy tonic, lubricates the intestines, is beneficial for constipation, and hastens the eruption of measles. These seeds go rancid quickly because of their high polyunsaturated fatty acid content. It is best to shell them before eating.

WALNUTS reduce inflammation and alleviate pain, due to a high content of Omega-3 oils. They moisten the lungs and intestines, help relieve coughing and wheezing, nourish the kidney-adrenals-brain, and enrich sperm. They are most beneficial for those with involuntary emission, impotency, painful back and knees, and constipation in the elderly. They may harbor parasites so it is best to roast them lightly before eating and store in the fridge.

HEALING PROPERTIES OF VEGETABLES

ASPARAGUS contains the diuretic asparagine, which helps to eliminate water through the kidneys. It is beneficial for those with kidney problems, but should not be used when there is inflammation. It also helps cleanse cholesterol from the arteries and is useful for those with hypertension and arteriosclerosis.

BEET strengthens the heart, improves circulation, purifies the blood, benefits the liver, is helpful for those with anemia, moistens the intestines, and promotes menstruation. For hormone regulation during menopause, use in conjunction with carrot and chlorophyll rich foods (greens) to impart hormone balance. Due to its rich silicon content it increases the body's ability to absorb calcium. It also helps those with liver stagnancy and liver ailments, as well as constipation, nervousness, and congestion of the vascular system.

BROCCOLI is a natural diuretic, brightens the eyes, and is useful for eye inflammation and near-sightedness. Broccoli contains high amounts of pantothenic acid and Vitamin A, aids weight loss, and helps to alleviate rough skin, cold sores, and other forms of herpes. It has more Vitamin C than citrus and is high in natural sulfur, iron, and B Vitamins, which build the immune system. Lightly cooked, broccoli will retain its rich chlorophyll content while activating the iron. The sulfur counteracts gas formation allowing you to absorb the iron.

CAULIFLOWER has similar healing properties to broccoli and cabbage. This cold weather crop is great for growing in winter and stores all winter long in cold cellars. The compound called indole-3-carbinol in cauliflower increases the activity of enzymes that break down and disable carcinogens (cancer-causing). This substance can affect the metabolism of estrogen in the body, and prevent breast and other female cancers. Cauliflower also detoxifies the system of the harmful forms of estrogen that result in reproductive cancers and complaints in women. Cauliflower contains allicin, which can improve heart health and reduce the risk of strokes, and selenium, a chemical that works well with Vitamin C to strengthen the immune system and maintain a healthy cholesterol level. It is an excellent source of vitamin A, B, and C, and of sulfur, fiber, potassium, and phosphorus.

CABBAGE moistens the intestines, benefits the stomach, improves digestion, and beautifies the skin. It is beneficial for those with constipation, the common cold, whooping cough (cabbage soup or tea), chronic cold feet, mental depression, and irritability. It also helps to rid the digestive system of worms (taken with garlic it is more effective against parasites), and purifies the blood. It contains Vitamin U, a remedy for either stomach or duodenal ulcers (drink 1 ½ cups of freshly made cabbage juice 2-3 times a day between meals for at least 2 weeks), and a good source of iodine and Vitamin C. Studies indicate that cruciferous vegetables such as cabbage, broccoli, and brussel sprouts inhibit cancerous growth in the large intestine.

CARROTS benefit the lungs, strengthen the spleen and pancreas, improve liver function, dissolve accumulations such as stones and tumors, help with indigestion, skin lesions, and heartburn, and eliminate putrefactive bacteria in the intestines that cause poor assimilation. Carrots are also effective for diarrhea, chronic dysentery, and destroying roundworm and pinworms in the intestines. Carrots are alkaline-forming and clear up acidic blood conditions including acne, tonsillitis, and rheumatism. They are protective against cancer, night blindness, ear infections, earaches, and deafness. Their large amount of beta-carotene and vitamins benefit the skin, lungs, digestive tract, and urinary tract infections. Carrots ease whooping cough and coughing in general. They also contain large amounts of silicon, thereby strengthening connective tissues and increasing ability to absorb and metabolize calcium.

CELERY improves digestion, purifies the blood, helps to control appetite, promotes sweating, and helps to clear digestive fermentation, rheumatism, arthritis, gout, and nerve inflammation. Helpful for blood in urine, burning when urinating, acne, and canker sores. It is a natural diuretic and high in potassium. Celery juice combined with lemon juice is a remedy for the common cold and headache and a good workout recovery drink. It is also very high in silicon that helps to renew joints, bones, arteries and all connective tissues. In food combining, celery goes well with fruit!

CHIVES influence repair in the kidneys, liver, and stomach. Chives increase circulation due to trauma, specifically for bruises, swelling, and other joint injuries. They strengthen the kidneys and sexual capacity making them beneficial for those with leukorrhea, urinary incontinence, spermatorrhea, and arthritic pain.
Note: Avoid chives when eye diseases and skin eruptions are present.

CUCUMBER is a natural diuretic that helps alleviate edema from the lower legs, cleanse the blood, counteract toxins, and lift depression. Cucumber is helpful for those with inflammatory conditions such as sore throat, acne, stomach inflammation, conjunctivitis, and discharge. It is a tonic for the heart, spleen-pancreas, stomach, and the large intestine. Cucumber quenches thirst, moistens lungs, purifies the skin and acts as a digestive aid. It is also high in erepsis, a digestive aid, which breaks down protein and cleanses the intestines enabling the body to destroy worms (especially tapeworms). Applied to the skin, it beautifies the complexion and relieves hot, inflamed, swollen, dry eyes.

EGGPLANT reduces swelling, clears stagnant blood, dissolves congealed blood specifically in the uterus and helps reduce excess bleeding. Eggplant is not good for pregnant mothers as it can cause miscarriages. It is used for conditions such as bleeding hemorrhoids, blood in the urine, dysentery, diarrhea, and canker sores (apply charred eggplant powder). Eggplant is also a rich source of bioflavonoid, which renews arteries, prevents strokes, and aids in calcium absorption. Eggplant aids cleansing of the liver and uterus and is particularly helpful for resolving repressed emotions and their harmful effects on these organs.

GARLIC promotes circulation and sweating, eliminates toxins from the body (including poison from heavy metals such as lead and mercury), removes abdominal obstructions, and inhibits the common cold virus as well as other viruses, amoebae, and other microorganisms. Garlic helps to eliminate worms, unfavorable bacteria, and yeast (Candida albican). It is also used for tuberculosis, asthma, hay fever, dysentery, Lyme disease, anthrax infection, warts, abscesses, and hepatitis. It is a remedy for colds, sore throats, and sinus headaches (hold a clove of garlic in the mouth for at least 15 minutes, and then consume it). To ward off mosquitoes, eat garlic at least once a day. For athlete's foot, sprinkle garlic powder on wet feet and let dry—socks may be worn. A drop of garlic in the ear canal once a day helps clear ear infections.
Note: Avoid using garlic when clearing the body of a fever but if taken early can halt a cold or flu.

JERUSALEM ARTICHOKE (SUNCHOKE) helps to relieve asthmatic conditions, cleanse the liver, significantly lowers blood LDL cholesterol levels, eases constipation, stimulates insulin production, and enhances athletic performance. It is loaded with potassium and has been known to effectively lower homocysteine levels. It contains inulin, which reduces insulin need, and is therefore highly beneficial for diabetics. If properly stored in the ground, it will keep for over 9 months.

KALE eases lung congestion, benefits the stomach, has natural anti-inflammatory properties and is great for anemic/weak persons. It is abundant in sulfur and can be used to help those with stomach and duodenal ulcers. Kale is an exceptional source of chlorophyll, amino acids, calcium, iron, and Vitamin A. In a 100 calorie portion, kale fulfills most of your recommended daily requirement for all vitamins and minerals.

KOHLRABI helps to increase circulation, eliminate blood coagulations, and calm indigestion and blood sugar imbalances. Those who are hypoglycemic and diabetic can use kohlrabi to good effect. Kohlrabi also relieves painful urination, stops bleeding in the colon, reduces swelling of the scrotum, and alleviates effects of intoxication from drugs and alcohol.

LEEK is helpful for those with dysphagia (difficulty swallowing), excess bleeding internally and externally, and diarrhea.

MUSHROOM helps to decrease fat levels in the blood, helps rid excess mucus in the lungs, has antibiotic properties, can aid in fighting contagious hepatitis, increases white blood cell count, has anti-tumor activity, can help stop post-surgery cancer metastasis, and promotes appetite.

MUSHROOM (SHIITAKE) is a natural source of interferon, a protein that appears to induce an immune response against cancers and viral diseases. It is used to help the body fight stomach and cervix cancers. These mushrooms also decrease both fat and cholesterol in the blood and help discharge the excess residues of accumulated animal protein.

MUSTARD GREENS benefit lung health for those who are susceptible to pneumonia or are smokers. Mustard greens also heal the intestines, clear chest congestion, improve energy circulation and reduce white copious mucus associated with lung infections. They are also used as a remedy for colds and coughs (simply pour boiling water over mustard greens and allow to steep for 10 minutes, then strain and drink the tea).
Note: Not good for those with inflamed eye disease or hemorrhoids.

ONION resolves sticky blood, therefore reducing the incidence of blood clotting. Onions help with frigidity (coldness), lower blood pressure, lower cholesterol, cleanse plaque in the arteries, and retard the growth of viruses, yeasts, ferments, and other pathogenic organisms. Onions are the richest food in sulfur, which helps purify the body, remove heavy metals and parasites, and facilitate protein/ amino acid metabolism. Eastern tradition holds that eating onions too often can foster excessive emotional desires.

PARSLEY improves digestion, detoxifies the body from meat or fish poisoning, ripens measles to hasten recovery, strengthens optic and brain nerves, strengthens adrenals, promotes urination, and is good for treating obesity and mucus in the bladder. Parsley contains an abundance of Vitamin C, A, chlorophyll, calcium, natural sodium, magnesium, and iron. Parsley is rich in Vitamin C and is thus a good blood cleanser. Raw parsley juice has some metabolic properties for the normal functioning of the adrenal and thyroid glands.
Note: Parsley should not be used by nursing mothers as it dries up milk production.

PARSNIP benefits spleen, pancreas and stomach health, helps clear liver and gall bladder obstructions, promotes perspiration, lubricates intestines (for those susceptible to constipation), acts as an analgesic, and is a source of concentrated silicon. Effective in soups or teas for cough, cold, shortness of breath, headaches, dizziness, rheumatism, and arthritis. *Note: Avoid parsnip leaves as they are poisonous.*

POTATO contains an abundance of sugar, potassium, and minerals, and neutralizes body acids, which help relieve arthritis and rheumatism. Potatoes are by nature alkaline-forming. If you are suffering from acid indigestion, potato juice can help to soak up the acid. You can make potato juice by washing organic potatoes and feeding them through a juicer. You may also peel them and soak in a cup of distilled water overnight, then drink the infused water the next day.

PUMPKIN relieves dysentery, eczema, and edema, helps regulate blood sugar imbalances, benefits pancreas health, and is used for diabetes and hypoglycemia. It also promotes discharge of mucus from the lungs, bronchi, and throat, and if used regularly helps benefit bronchial asthma. Cooked pumpkin destroys intestinal worms, but not as effectively as the pumpkin seed.

RADISH moistens the lungs, cuts mucus, detoxifies the body, and clears sinus congestion, hoarseness, phlegm, and sore throats. Radish helps cleanse the gallbladder, relieving indigestion and abdominal swelling. The toxin purging property of the radish makes it useful for detoxifying old residues in the body during healthy diet upgrades.

ROMAINE LETTUCE dries up damp conditions in the body such as edema, digestive ferments and yeasts. It is helpful in overcoming hemorrhoids, acts as a natural diuretic, and alleviates scant urine and blood in urine. It is one of the highest sources of silicon in vegetables, which allows the body to metabolize and absorb calcium effectively. Lettuce is also used for increasing mother's milk production.

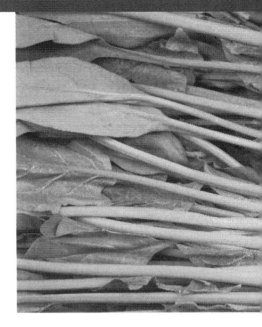

SPINACH builds the blood, stops bleeding, is a natural laxative and diuretic, builds red blood cells for those with anemia, quenches thirst, and cleanses the blood of toxins that cause skin disease. Spinach can assist in ridding the body of constipation and urinary difficulty. Due to its high sulfur content it relieves herpes irritations. Spinach is also good for improving night blindness. *Note: All leafy greens combine well with fruits of all varieties for efficient digestion.*

SCALLION is used in cases of both chest and heart pain. Scallions promote urination and sweating and relieve edema, diarrhea, abdominal swelling/pain, and arthritis.
Note: Avoid if you have yellow mucus, fever, and great thirst.

SQUASH is healing for stomach, spleen, and pancreas ailments. It reduces inflammations and burns (fresh squash juice is applied to the burn), improves circulation, and alleviates pain. Summer squashes and zucchini help overcome summer heat, water retention/edema, and difficulty urinating. Steamed summer squash or zucchini with its skin and seeds destroys worms in the colon.

SWEET POTATO & YAM strengthen the spleen and pancreas, increase milk in lactating mothers, remove toxins from the body, aid kidney function, and treat thinness and diarrhea. These root vegetables are rich in Vitamin A, which is helpful for night blindness. Spirulina and organic animal liver added to sweet potato soups make a highly effective night-blindness formula. Because they're rich in fiber, yams fill you up without filling out your hips and waistline. Yams are also a good source of manganese, a trace mineral that helps with carbohydrate metabolism and is a cofactor in a number of enzymes important in energy production and antioxidant defenses.

TOMATO relieves thirst, strengthens the health of the stomach, cleanses the liver, purifies the blood, detoxifies the body, encourages digestion, and helps with diminished appetite. It also alleviates indigestion, food retention in the colon, anorexia, constipation, high blood pressure, red eyes, and headache. Tomato is alkalinizing, reducing acidic blood for those dealing with rheumatism and gout. Large amounts of tomato weaken everyone, and should be avoided by those with arthritis.

TURNIP improves circulation, detoxifies the body, builds red blood cells, resolves mucus conditions in nose and lungs, relieves coughing, clears food stagnancies in the stomach, and improves appetite. Turnip is generally helpful for indigestion, hoarseness, diabetes, and jaundice. Turnip works best when used in its raw state.

WATERCRESS aids healing and protection for the lungs, stomach, bladder, and kidneys. It is a diuretic, purifies the blood, removes stagnant blood, helps reduce cancerous growths, benefits night vision, and clears facial blemishes. Watercress is a rich source of Vitamin A, chlorophyll, sulfur, and calcium. It also helps to dry up and eliminate yellow phlegm due to flu and colds.

HEALING PROPERTIES OF HERBS & SPICES

ANISE has gas prevention properties, aids in digestion, is diuretic, improves eyesight, refreshes mouth and removes bad smell, helps the bowels to expel fecal matter, and relieves pain in joints. Boil approximately six grams of aniseeds in water, let cool, and bottle it thereafter. Infusion of aniseeds with unrefined cane sugar or honey will regulate menses. Take 5-6 grams of aniseeds to improve liver functioning and eyesight, as well as to restore equilibrium.

BASIL is an antidepressant, antiseptic, adrenal stimulant, digestive, and anti-parasitic, and combats fevers and headaches. Containing properties similar to aspirin, basil also exhibits anti-inflammatory properties, making it a good food to consume by people who have problems with arthritis. An oil in basil called eugenol blocks the activity of an enzyme in the body called cyclooxygenase. This enzyme normally causes swelling and pain. For respiratory disorders make a tea or decoction of the leaves and add honey and ginger. This is an effective remedy for bronchitis, asthma, influenza, cough, and cold. A decoction of the leaves, cloves, and common salt also gives immediate relief in case of influenza. Leaves should be boiled in half a liter of water until half the water has dissipated, then drink mixture.

BAMBOO manna, dried sugar-like granules found in many varieties of bamboo, acts as an aphrodisiac and a diuretic and lowers fever. To eliminate worm infestations, dissolve pieces of bamboo manna in warm water and add a few crushed cumin seeds to it. Take this preparation daily for a couple weeks to dislodge and expel worms. Bamboo manna is also a highly useful expectorant, stopping and soothing coughs. Simply mix some powdered manna with honey and lick off the spoon. Its properties soothe lung tissue. You can obtain this food online or at a local Asian market.

BLACK PEPPER has anti-diarrheal properties and acts as a natural antibacterial and circulatory stimulant. To relieve even chronic diarrhea, one teaspoonful of fine powdered pepper should be taken with water. To relieve inflammation, use finely powdered pepper and salt and massage over the gums. For painful joints, mix equal parts black pepper, cumin, and ginger boiled in mustard oil for an effective massage oil. *Note: Avoid black pepper if you have fungal or Candida infections.*

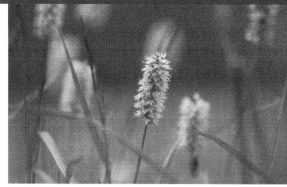

BISTORT extracts are used to stop external and internal bleeding. Bistort has been used externally for hemorrhoids, insect bites, measles, snakebites, and small burns or wounds; as a mouthwash or gargle for canker sores, gum problems, laryngitis, and sore throat; and to reduce pulmonary secretions. Internally, bistort has been used to treat dysentery, gastric and pulmonary hemorrhage, irritable bowel syndrome, jaundice, peptic ulcers, and ulcerative colitis. It has also been used as an anthelmintic, an antidote for certain poisons, and a douche for excessive vaginal discharge or bleeding. The 1983 British Herbal Pharmacopoeia reports that bistort exerts an anti-inflammatory activity and lists it as useful in treating diarrhea in children.

CARDAMOM is used for its carminative, stimulant, laxative, detoxifying, and vitalizing properties. It boosts digestion and combats flatulence. Chewing on cardamom is effectively used to eliminate colic and headaches. It effectively arrests nausea, vomiting, stomach pain, and phlegm. It is recommend to be eaten along with honey for improving eyesight. Cardamom is also excellent for detoxifying the body against the toxic effects of caffeine and mucus-forming foods. It is also an excellent remedy for hiccups. You can use the essential oil of cardamom in warm water as a gargle for combating halitosis (bad breath). Cardamom tea is used in various parts of the world to refresh the mind and body and also for treating respiratory tract infections such as cold and cough. This warm aromatic herb has excellent tonic and stimulating properties and is widely used in Europe and the Middle East to flavor coffee, curries, confectioneries, and wine. The essential oil of cardamom is used for boosting digestion and is known to possess powerful aphrodisiac qualities. It combats nausea and reduces the symptoms caused by PMS. It also treats cough and keeps the body warm. Monoterpenes is a substance found in cardamom oil that has potent antibacterial, antiviral, and antimycotic properties inhibiting the growth of fungi. Cardamom sprinkled on cooked cereal has been reported to help children with celiac disease (intolerance to gluten).

CAYENNE PEPPER increases circulation and is antifungal and antibacterial. Open up nasal passages and reduce swollen membranes by blending ginger and cayenne pepper together with honey in 6-8 oz. of warm water, then drink slowly. Chile peppers, especially hotter varieties such as Cayenne and Habanero, can be used externally as a remedy for joint pain, frostbite, and uncontrolled bleeding from a cut. The capsicum in the pepper stimulates blood flow to the affected area, which helps to reduce inflammation and discomfort. Sprinkle a little powder into gloves or shoes to help stimulate circulation and keep the hands and feet warm. To make a liniment for external use, gently boil one tablespoon of hot pepper in one pint of cider vinegar. Do not strain, and bottle while still hot. Spices, especially ginger and cayenne pepper, increase circulation and improve blood flow to stiff, sore areas, easing the pain of aching muscles.

CELERY & CELERY SEED is very effective for diseases arising from acidity and toxemia, rheumatism and gout. It reduces fluid retention and arthritic conditions and aids urinary and kidney function. It is useful in the treatment of arthritis due to its high sodium content. Its organic sodium tends to prevent and relieve deposits in the joints. For optimum results, it should be taken in the form of freshly extracted juice, made with the leaves as well as the stem. For gout and rheumatism, use the fluid extract of the seeds or celery seed sprout, as it is more powerful than the raw celery plant. Its regular use prevents stone formation in the gall bladder and kidneys. The herb is valuable in diseases of the blood such as anemia, leukemia, Hodgkin's disease, purpura and hemophilia caused by the inorganic mineral elements and salts taken into the body by means of devitalized foods and sedatives. This plant is very high in magnesium and iron content, a combination which is invaluable as a food for the blood cells. The juice of celery in combination with carrot juice should be taken for the treatment of these disorders.

CHILI PEPPER is antibacterial and serves as a digestive aid. It relieves symptoms from colds, sore throats and fevers, and improves circulation, especially for cold hands and feet, and is useful as a hangover remedy. It works to resolve the symptoms of Emphysema within one month. Include five to eight chili peppers (encapsulated) in your daily diet. Peppers can act as a heart stimulant to reduce or eliminate heart attacks by regulating blood flow while strengthening the integrity of arterial walls. Nutritionally, fresh chili peppers are an excellent source of calcium and Vitamin C, and are also known to reduce sinusitis, enhance skin elasticity, and strengthen the immune system. You can make a chili pepper tincture, especially from the hottest varieties, by drying the peppers and grinding into a powder. Use one or two tablespoons in warm water for the relief of many symptoms. For a more convenient method, pack chili powder into gel capsules instead of taking in tea form. To calm down severe toothaches, press out fresh chili pepper oil. Using a garlic press, and placing a small piece of cheese cloth inside the press, slowly extract about _ teaspoon of chili oil. Put the oil on half a cotton ball (or the cotton from the end of a Q-tip®) and press into the affected tooth cavity.

CINNAMON balances blood sugar, possesses antibacterial, antifungal, and antiviral properties, and improves circulation. Cinnamon is widely used as an efficient herbal remedy for reducing arthritic pain. Take half a teaspoonful of cinnamon powder and add in one teaspoonful honey, and take this combination in the morning on an empty stomach. Positive results will be visible within one week. For those with Type 2 diabetes, use this remedy: in the morning, on an empty stomach, consume _ teaspoon cinnamon powder and 1 tsp. Agave nectar mixed in _ glass of lukewarm water. For cluster headaches and migraines, make a fine paste of cinnamon powder and water and apply this on the forehead.

Note: Be careful to purchase only true cinnamon from the bark of a cinnamon tree and not the more common "cinnamon" from the bark of the cassia tree (which is cheaper and more widely available).

CLOVES stop nausea, aid digestion, and support the reproductive organs and kidneys. Cloves are also used to reduce gum irritation and inflammation.

CORIANDER helps in the digestion of legumes, aids in balancing blood sugar levels, and possesses anti-inflammatory properties. It is also antimicrobial and possesses anxiety-lowering and cholesterol-lowering effects.

CUMIN is high in iron and acts as a digestive aid, aiding in liver detoxification. It is rich in thymol and possesses anti-parasitic properties targeting hookworm infections, and also serves as an antiseptic in many proprietary preparations. It is a stimulant, which increases the secretion and discharge of urine, and relieves flatulence. It strengthens the functions of the stomach and arrests any bleeding. For amnesia or dullness of memory, mix three grams of ground black cumin seed with 12 grams of pure honey. Eat one tablespoon two times a day.

DILL helps eliminate flatulence and digestive disturbances, has anticancer and antimicrobial effects, and promotes liver detoxification.

EUCALYPTUS has been shown to exert antifungal, anti-inflammatory, and antimicrobial effects. Warning: Eucalyptus oil may not be safe for patients receiving hypoglycemic therapy or for pregnant or breast-feeding mothers.

fennel

FENNEL aids bean digestion, is anti-inflammatory, soothes digestive upset, is a circulatory stimulant, stimulates milk flow in nursing mothers, and encourages mental alertness.

FENUGREEK soothes inflamed stomach and intestines and cleanses the stomach, bowels, kidneys and respiratory tract from excess mucus. It is also useful in the healing of peptic ulcers because it forms a healthy coating of mucilaginous matter as a protective layer. Fenugreek seeds made into tea are just as effective as quinine in reducing fevers. Fenugreek can normalize a woman's system after delivering a baby. Drink plenty of fenugreek water (a teaspoon of seed soaked in a pint of water overnight) during the early stages of small pox/chicken pox or measles. The alkaloid trigonelline in fenugreek is antiseptic and carminative. For preventing joint stiffness, drink one teaspoon of fenugreek powder in some warm water. Fenugreek seeds are very useful in diabetes. Soak about 90-100 seeds in 250 grams of water and leave it overnight. Mash them in the morning, strain, and drink the mixture regularly. You can also add fenugreek seeds to soups and salads.

GINGER calms upset stomach and increases circulation to lower extremities. It protects the intestinal lining against ulceration and has a wide range of actions against intestinal parasites. For indigestion, use a decoction of 1/2 teaspoon dry ginger and 1/8 teaspoon rock salt in warm water. For jaundice, take one teaspoon of dry ginger powder with some honey or raw cane sugar twice a day for smooth bowel movements and as a liver tonic. To make ginger tea, add crushed ginger to boiling water and let it simmer 20 minutes to decrease inflammation and relieve congestion and body aches. For asthma, add a few garlic cloves to the above tea. To relieve chest congestion, mix ginger with mustard oil and apply externally on the chest. For blood in the urine, boil one teaspoon of dry ginger in eight ounces of milk and drink twice a day. For use on stings, use dry ginger paste mixed in yogurt as an effective topical application to reduce the swelling. For scrotal swelling, apply a mixture of dry ginger and salt solution to reduce pain and swelling. For earaches, crush or press 1/4 inch ginger to get fresh juice, warm up a little, and place a few drops in the ear to relieve pain and clear infected area.

HONEY is known to increase blood flow to the heart, soothe and tranquilize agitated and tense nerves, lower blood pressure, add weight to thin persons, ease coughs, impart strength to lungs, quench thirst, remove dryness of mouth, and help with sinusitis and breathing problems. For weight loss, take this mixture in the morning on an empty stomach: honey and lemon juice or apple cider vinegar mixed in lukewarm water.

LEMON BALM improves circulation, provides headache relief, is an antidepressant, digestive stimulant, is antibacterial, antiviral, and helps with anxiety and headache relief.

learn more at
**www.herbwisdom.com/
herb-licorice-root.html**

LICORICE is antispasmodic, anti-tussive (stops coughing), relieves constipation and gastric ulcers, is anti-allergenic, improves adrenal function, is laxative, and reduces pain in the body. It has also been used for many ailments including asthma, athlete's foot, baldness, body odor, bursitis, canker sores, chronic fatigue, depression, colds and flu, coughs, dandruff, emphysema, gingivitis and tooth decay, gout, heartburn, HIV, viral infections, fungal infections, ulcers, liver problems, Lyme disease, menopause, psoriasis, shingles, sore throat, tendinitis, tuberculosis, ulcers, yeast infections, prostate enlargement, and arthritis. It also mimics the behavior of corticosteroids when used for relieving an allergic reaction.
Note: Avoid if you have high blood pressure.

MARJORAM is antimicrobial, kills amoebas, inhibits growth of bacteria, and serves as an antioxidant. It is similar to oregano in character.

NUTMEG improves appetite, provides migraine relief, helps with nausea, reduces abdominal bloating, indigestion, colic, and is anti-inflammatory. Mix together 1/4 teaspoon ground up nutmeg with honey or a small amount of mashed up bananas.

ORANGE OIL is anti-inflammatory, anti-spasmodic, anti-diar-rhea, and anti-depressant.

For more on oils visit
www.organicfacts.net

OREGANO consists of volatile oils that inhibit the growth of bacteria, candida, and other parasitic microorganisms. Some studies found this medicinal herb to be more effective in killing Giardia (infection of the small intestine) than prescription drugs. Oregano supplements are also used for external and internal fungal infections. Externally, pound a handful of fresh oregano leaves into a paste (adding a small amount of hot water, tea, or oatmeal to reach desired consistency), then use the paste to relieve pain from rheumatism, swelling, itching, aching muscles, and sores. For tired joints and muscles, take a bath in oregano: place a handful of oregano leaves in a cheesecloth bag or coffee filter under steaming bath water, then allow it to steep in the tub with you as you relax in the warm, fragrant water. For arthritis and rheumatism, rub oil of oregano on affected joints in the morning and before bedtime until the condition improves. For angina chest pain, take two drops of garlic oil with five drops of oregano oil with coconut milk or plain yogurt.

PAPRIKA improves blood circulation, reduces indigestion, aids stomach ulcers, aids heartburn, and helps combat colds and sinus infections.

PEPPERMINT cools the body from heat conditions, aids digestion, reduces flatulence, is a diaphoretic, and reduces nausea and motion sickness. This herb is useful for calming the nervous system, upset stomach, respiratory conditions such as colds, coughing, acute respiratory difficulties, and for bacteria, fungal, and viral infections. Peppermint has also been used to reduce muscle spasms associated with endoscopy, colonoscopy, and barium enemas. *Note: DO NOT use on children under four.*

ROSEMARY brings oxygen directly to the brain, aids digestion, relieves flatulence, headache/migraine, and indigestion, is used to darken graying hair, and is anti-dandruff. Rosemary tea is also used for colic, colds, and may lift nervous depression.

SPEARMINT is similar in use and function to peppermint. Please see peppermint for details.

TARRAGON is antifungal, antimicrobial, and antioxidant, benefits diabetics, reduces the desire to overeat, and aids weight loss.

rosemary

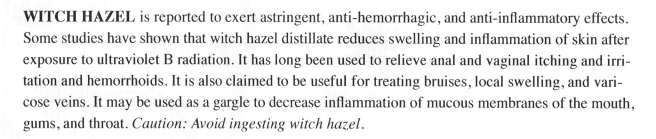

TURMERIC soothes joints, is antioxidant, aids injury recovery, improves flexibility, reduces LDL cholesterol levels, improves skin, improves blood flow (which can reduce blood pressure), reduces pain, and is a natural antibiotic. It relieves intestinal gas by reducing gas-forming bacteria, has antifungal activity, and has been traditionally used for relieving inflammation.

Warning: Turmeric should not be taken if you have a bile duct blockage, a blood-clotting disorder, or stomach ulcers (or a history of them). Pregnant and nursing women should use discretion in using turmeric, as the effects in such cases are unknown.

THYME aids digestion, clears phlegm, combats chest infections, is antimicrobial, antispasmodic, antibiotic, and heals wounds.

SAGE is antispasmodic (calms nerves and muscles), has a high estrogen content, is antioxidant, hypoglycemic, works as a uterine stimulant, suppresses perspiration, and heals mucus membranes.

SEA SALT is naturally high in minerals, making it a good source of natural iodine and trace minerals. It sterilizes cuts and neutralizes pain from bee stings and bug bites.

WHITE PEPPER is a digestive aid and soothes the stomach.

WITCH HAZEL is reported to exert astringent, anti-hemorrhagic, and anti-inflammatory effects. Some studies have shown that witch hazel distillate reduces swelling and inflammation of skin after exposure to ultraviolet B radiation. It has long been used to relieve anal and vaginal itching and irritation and hemorrhoids. It is also claimed to be useful for treating bruises, local swelling, and varicose veins. It may be used as a gargle to decrease inflammation of mucous membranes of the mouth, gums, and throat. *Caution: Avoid ingesting witch hazel.*

MAKE FOOD INTO HEALING TEAS

Congee Tea is known in Eastern medicine as "Tea for Healing." This tea is a thin porridge of rice that can be mixed with other grains, beans, vegetables, or herbs. It is best to drink three cups of congee tea a day for chronic conditions and then reduce to one time a day for maintenance. To make the tea, measure out 6 cups of water, one handful of brown rice, and your ingredient of choice and put in a crock-pot or covered pot. You can mix and match various herbs with the base ingredients listed on the next page to make your own healing tea.

What is the right measurement of the extra ingredients for the tea? For beans use one handful, for vegetables use 4 cups, and for herbs and seeds use 2-5 tablespoons. Cook the congee tea four to six hours at the lowest temperature possible. It should end up being a thick drink the consistency of porridge; you may strain it or drink it all together. It is better to use more water than not enough, so add water if it you feel it is too thick for your liking. This is a short list of the foods that can be made into congee tea. You can use other foods and herbs that are listed in the Healing Properties of Foods section.

Aduki Bean: A natural diuretic, curative for swelling, edema, and gout.

Carrot: Digestive aid; eliminates flatulence.

Celery: Cooling in summer; benefits large intestine.

Chestnut: Strengthens kidneys, knees and loin; useful in treating anal hemorrhages.

Fennel: Harmonizes the stomach, expels gas, and heals hernias.

Ginger: Used for digestive weakness: diarrhea, anorexia, vomiting, and indigestion.

Mung Bean: Reduces fevers; a food for summer heat; relieves thirst.

Mustard: Expels phlegm; clears stomach congestion.

Purslane: Detoxifies body, recommended for rheumatism and swellings.

Sweet Brown Rice: Used for diarrhea, vomiting, and indigestion.

Sesame Seed: Lubricates intestines, helps those with rheumatism.

Rye: Helpful for easing migraine headaches.

Taro Root: Aids stomach, builds blood, and good for those who are anemic.

REMEDIES AND GUIDELINES FOR YOUR DISEASE

Taking responsibility for your health is both freeing and empowering! You can make your own home remedies and natural cures at home from natural ingredients such as fruits, vegetables, and herbs. Use this section as a starting point for creating a lifestyle that can resolve physical problems. The suggestions below can be fully or partially applied to your lifestyle. The more changes you make to your current situation, the faster the results. For those with sensitive systems, be cautious of over-loading or detoxing the body too quickly. A good tip is to start in two's: add two foods, avoid two foods, and take two herbs. Then allow your body some time to get acquainted with the changes before you implement more. Within a week you should begin to see improvement. Take the time to journal and record any changes you experience, both positive and negative, and adjust accordingly.

Think of your body as a house. When you move out you create a huge mess at first, but once you have packed up everything, you follow up with a deep cleaning and then the new tenant can move in. Many times you have to agitate your body systems before you see results. Results are not measured by how you feel during the cleanup process but in the final outcome.

The healing nature of foods and herbs offers subtle yet long-lasting benefits, with little or no side effects. Give yourself time to see and respond to results before jumping back onto the medical bandwagon.

PMS

Foods to Eat	Foods to Avoid	Herbs	Nutritional Support
Green leafy vegetables	Red meats	Red raspberry leaf	Vita Synergy
Fruits	Dairy	Angelica root	Stinging Nettles
Wild caught salmon	Sugars	Blessed thistle	Sea Minerals
Chia seed	Processed foods	Sarsaparilla root	Probiotic
Wheat germ	Fast foods	Milk thistle	Bone Response
Brewer's yeast	Salt	Wild yam extract	Blue Green Algae
Raw cocoa nibs	Alcohol	Corn silk	Spirulina
Sprouted grains	Trans-fatty acids	Primrose oil	
Brown rice	Caffeine		
Avocado			
Flax seed			
Mung beans			

SEASONAL ALLERGIES AND HAY FEVER

Foods to Eat	Foods to Avoid	Herbs	Nutritional Support
Horseradish	Breads & cake	Alfalfa	Bromelain
Kale	Coffee	Nettle leaf	Healing Honey
Cod liver oil	Chocolate	Eucalyptus oil	Quercetin
Fresh garlic	Dairy	Yarrow extract	Vita Synergy
Fresh vegetables	Sugar	Goldenseal *(use for*	Radiance C powder
Fresh fruits	Soft drinks	*only 7 days)*	Stinging Nettle
Raw nuts and seeds	White flour		Sea Minerals
Ground chia seed			

RHEUMATOID ARTHRITIS

Foods to Eat	Foods to Avoid	Herbs	Nutritional Support
Ground chia seed	Meats	Boswellia	Pure Synergy
Herring	Sugars	Bromelain	Sea Minerals
Salmon	Omega-6 fatty acids	Cat's claw	Zrii
Kale	Agrimony	Cayenne	Radiance C powder
Ginger	Siberian ginseng	Alfalfa	
Barley grass	Breads & cake		
Broccoli	Coffee		
Dark leafy greens	Chocolate		
	Dairy		
	Sugar		
	Soft drinks		
	White flour		

Consume Healing Foods--Avoid Deceptive Foods

OSTEOARTHRITIS

Foods to Eat	Foods to Avoid	Herbs	Nutritional Support
Blackstrap molasses	All dairy	Alfalfa	Food Derived Vit. C
Fresh pineapple	All meat	Ashwaganda	Barley Life
Dark leafy greens	Citrus fruit	Boswellia	Leafy Greens
Kale	Breads & pastries	Cat's claw	Turmeric
Broccoli	Coffee & caffeine	Hawthorn	Innate Calcium
Cabbage	Chocolate	Tumeric	
Ginger	Sugar		
Oats	Soft drinks		
Cherries	White flour		
Sprouts	Wheat flour		
Sprouted grain bread			

OSTEOPOROSIS, OSTEOPENIA

Foods to Eat	Foods to Avoid	Herbs	Nutritional Support
Kale	Yeast	Alfalfa	Zrii
Cabbage	Breads & pastries	Feverfew	Bone Response
Broccoli	Coffee & caffeine	Hawthorn	(Innate™)
Spinach	Chocolate	Coleus	Hawthorn Sea
Blueberries	Sugar		Minerals
Garlic	Soft drinks		Radiance C powder
Onions	White flour		Pure Synergy Greens
Oats	Wheat flour		Barley Greens
Cherries	Fried foods		
Brown rice	All meat		
Black beans			
Wild caught salmon			
Raw goat's milk			
Raw goat's cheese			

HYPOTHYROIDISM

Foods to Eat	Foods to Avoid	Herbs	Nutritional Support
Kelp	Breads & pastries	Bayberry	BioAge Superfood
Nori	Coffee & caffeine	Black cohosh	Pure Synergy Greens
Dulse	Chocolate	Goldenseal *(use for*	Klamath Krystals
Salmon	Sugar	*only 7 days)*	Ioderal
Walnuts	Soft drinks	Gentian	
Pumpkin seeds	White flour	Mugwort	
Dates	Wheat flour	Primrose	
Parsley	Fried foods		
Molasses	All meat	Oils:	
	Gluten	Geranium	
	MSG	Jasmine	
	Tap water		

LUPUS

Foods to Eat	Foods to Avoid	Herbs	Nutritional Support
Raw vegetables	Breads & pastries	Alfalfa	Supa Boost Sea Minerals
Brown rice	Coffee & caffeine	Feverfew	
Salmon	Chocolate	Pau d'arco	Zrii
Wheat germ	Sugar	Red clover	Pure Synergy Greens
Olive oil	Soft drinks	Milk thistle	Barley Life
Onions	White flour	Yucca	Just Carrots
Garlic	Wheat flour	Chinese Licorice	Protolytic Enzymes
Fresh pineapple	Fried foods	Primrose oil	Radiance C powder
	All meat		Antioxidant
	Gluten		BioAge Superfood
	MSG		Undenatured Whey
	Tap water		Protein

IRRITABLE BOWEL SYNDROME

Foods to Eat	Foods to Avoid	Herbs	Nutritional Support
Brown rice	Wheat	Milk thistle extract	Probiotic
Legumes	Sugar	Slippery elm	Kyolic (garlic)
Raw vegetables	Red meat	Primrose oil	Vita Synergy
Sauerkraut	Dairy	Pau d'arco	Russian Choice GI
Goat Yogurt		Chinese licorice	Zrii
Goat Kefir		Alfalfa	Digestive Enzymes
Fresh fruits		Aloe vera juice	
Brewer's yeast		Peppermint	

HEADACHES: MIGRAINES, CLUSTER, TENSION

Foods to Eat	Foods to Avoid	Herbs	Nutritional Support
Green leafy vegetables	Foods containing tyramine	Cayenne	Supa Boost Sea Minerals
Beans	Cheese	Chamomile	Vita Synergy
Nuts	Chocolate	Gingko biloba	Pure Synergy Greens
Wheat germ	Coffee	Jamaica dogweed (sinus)	Barley Life
Salmon	Alcohol	Kava kava (tension)	Zrii
Ginger	Dairy	White willow (bark)	
		Peppermint	
		Valerian root	

FOOD POISONING

Foods to Eat	Foods to Avoid	Herbs	Nutritional Support
Water	Dairy	*Sooth digestion:*	Reishi mushrooms
Soup	Fats	Ginger	Oregano oil
Broths	Oils	Aloe vera juice	
Steamed veggies	Sugar	Peppermint	
Brown rice	Caffeine	Fennel tea & seed	
Garlic	Alcohol		
Fresh apple,		*Kill the poison:*	
carrot, celery juice		Arsenicum album	
		Activated charcoal	
		Wormwood	
		Goldenseal tea	
		Clove	
		Milk thistle	
		Lobelia	
		Activated Charcoal	

Caution: If you have any suspicion of food poisoning, contact your physician immediately.
Food poisoning is most commonly a reaction to toxins produced by bacteria, chemicals, heavy metals, parasites, fungi, or viruses found in raw foods like meat, fish, seafood, or foods that were contaminated by them.

Infants, older persons, women who are pregnant, and anyone with a compromised immune system are especially susceptible to food-borne illness. These people should never consume raw fish, raw seafood, or raw meat type products.

Consume Healing Foods--Avoid Deceptive Foods

HERPES

Foods to Eat	Foods to Avoid	Herbs	Nutritional Support
Goat yogurt	Peanuts	Astragalus	Pure Synergy Greens
Bell peppers	Brazil nuts	Acerola	Zrii
Beets	Pine nuts	Cat's claw	L-Lysine
Carrots & collards	Walnuts	Clove	Vitamin C
Brussels sprouts	Meat	Sage	Zinc
Broccoli & cabbage	Almonds	Lemon balm extract	Bee Pollen
Mustard	Wheat	Bee propolis	
Avocado	Chocolate	Aloe (externally)	
Strawberries	Sugars	Cayenne (externally)	
Apples & mangos	Tomatoes	Green tea compress	
Elderberries	Citrus fruits	Licorice root	
Legumes			

WARTS

Foods to Eat	Foods to Avoid	Herbs	Nutritional Support
Garlic	Sugars	Aloe vera	Radiance C
Fresh vegetables	Pork	Thuja	Zrii
Fresh fruits	Alcohol	Olive leaf extract	Barley Life
Whole foods	White & wheat bread	Echinacea	Liquid Kyolic
Brazil nuts		Astragalus	Selenium
Brewer's Yeast		Black walnut	Vitamin B-1,B12
Green tea extract		Blood root	Zinc
Bee propolis			
Bee pollen		*Topical Use:*	
		Garlic	
		Tea tree oil	

NOTE: Warts are common, contagious, and are caused by a viral infection, specifically by the aerobic Human Papilloma Virus (HPV). They typically disappear after a few months but can last for years and can recur. A few Papilloma viruses are known to cause cancer.

ULCERS

Foods to Eat	Foods to Avoid	Herbs	Nutritional Support
Apples	Sugar	Chinese licorice	Probiotic
Oats	Spicy foods	Mastic gum	Radiance C
Green leafy vegetables	Citrus fruits	Slippery elm	Chia Seeds
Cabbage juice	Coffee	Goldenseal (only 7 day	Vitamin A
Goat yogurt	Black tea	use)	Zinc
Bananas	Alcohol	Chamomile	
Blueberries	Salt animal fats	Aloe vera juice	
Artichoke		Cloves	
Cinnamon			
Pumpkin seeds			
Kefir			
Green tea			
Garlic w/ meals			

GOUT

Foods to Eat	Foods to Avoid	Herbs	Nutritional Support
Chia Seed	All meat	Celery seed extract	Fish oil
Flax Seed	All cow dairy	Nettle root	Chia seed
	Mushrooms	Chlorella	Probiotic
Fresh veggie juices:	Eggs	Bilberry	Digestive enzymes
Broccoli, Celery,	Peas	Bromelain	Zyphlamend
Lettuce, Beets, Kale,	Lentils	Sarsaparilla	Zrii
Parsley	Shellfish	Boswellia	Turmeric Force
	Asparagus	Turmeric	Rose hip tea
Fresh fruit & juices:	Sugar	Uva Ursi	Borage oil
Apples	Dried fruits		
Cherries	Beer		
Papaya	Alcohol		
Pineapple	Wheat gluten		
Blueberries	Roasted nuts		
Lemons			

HEMORRHOIDS

Foods to Eat	Foods to Avoid	Herbs	Nutritional Support
Raw fruits	Fried foods	Aloe Vera	Synergy greens
Raw vegetables	Caffeine	Calendula	Radiance C
Legumes & beans	Alcohol	Butcher's broom	Probiotics
Sesame seeds	Sugars	St. John's wart	Hem-Soothe
Prunes	Spicy foods	Horse chestnut	Zrii
Red palm oil	Dairy	Collinsonia	Rutin
Coconut kefir	Wheat	Witch hazel	Vitamin E
Goat yogurt	Citrus fruits	Horsetail	
Wheat germ	Peanuts	Bilberry	Dietary Fiber
Berries			Chia seeds
		Directly Apply:	Flax seeds
Fresh juices:		Plantain	Psyllium
Kale		Peruvian balsam	Pectin
Leafy greens		Witch hazel	

CANCER

Foods to Eat	Foods to Avoid	Herbs	Nutritional Support
Chia seeds	Fried foods	Black cohosh	Zrii
Dark leafy greens	Processed foods	Turmeric	Pure Synergy Greens
Raw vegetables	Junk food	Melatonin	Vita-Synergy
Raw fruits	Sugars	Milk thistle	Radiance C
Asparagus	Red meat	Cat's claw	Chia Seeds
Avocados	Caffeine	Pau d'arco	Probiotic
Cabbage, broccoli	Alcohol	Graviola	Maitaki Gold
Carrots	Spicy foods		
Garlic & onions	Dairy		
Organic berries	Wheat		
Wheat germ	Dried fruit		
Green tea	Coffee		
Brown rice	Butter		
	Soy & corn		

This entire book was designed to help your body eliminate the disease within so you can live. Follow the book's guidelines, apply the actions, and you will see your disease fall away. Doing the work halfway will not give you the results; follow the plan correctly and you will have success!

FIBROMYALGIA

Foods to Eat	Foods to Avoid	Herbs	Nutritional Support
Raw vegetables	Caffeine	Hydroxytryptophan	Magnesium
Leafy greens	Meat	Malic acid	Enzymes
Beans	Fried foods	Acidophilus	Radiance C
Raw nuts	Dairy products	Coenzyme Q-10	
Salmon	Sugar	Lecithin	
Pomegranates	Processed foods		
Kefir	Carbonated drinks		
Flax seed	Wheat		
Kelp			
Almonds			
Broccoli			

COLDS & FLU

Foods to Eat	Foods to Avoid	Herbs	Nutritional Support
Chicken & vegetable soup	All dairy	Cat's claw	Oil of oregano
Garlic	Sugar	Echinacea tea	Radiance C
Cabbage	Coffee	Fresh ginger root tea	Olive leaf extract
Whole green peppers	Black teas	Elderberry	Maca Root
Parsley	Chocolate	Chamomile	Zrii
Carrots	Muffins	Cayenne red pepper	Barley or wheat grass
Broccoli	Fried foods	Peppermint	Pure Synergy Super-food
Turnips		Anise	
Parsnips			
Lemon juice			
Grapefruits			

Consume Healing Foods--Avoid Deceptive Foods

FEVER

Foods to Eat	Foods to Avoid	Herbs	Nutritional Support
Papaya juice	Sugar	*Enhances use of herbs:*	Vitamin C
Water	Heavy meals	Aloe vera juice	Aecorola
Ginger tea	Soda		Zrii
Raw honey	Caffeine	*Breaks fever:*	Omega's
Apple cider vinegar	Alcohol	Echinacea tincture	
	Dairy	Catnip	
Juices:	All processed foods	Sage	
Fresh citrus fruits, especially oranges			
		Lowers temperature:	
Promotes sweating:		Hyssop, thyme, licorice	
Cayenne & garlic		White willow bark	
Soup w/ chili, cayenne		Chamomile	
Ginger tea		Peppermint	
		Spearmint	
		Fenugreek	

NOTE: *At the onset of fever it is best to eliminate all solid foods and drink lots of liquids. Lemon juice water and raw honey will cleanse the body. Use spicy soups or broths (unless fever is accompanied by nausea, then just use the Herbal Remedies) to encourage sweating, which cools the body.*

MENOPAUSE

Foods to Eat	Foods to Avoid	Herbs	Nutritional Support
Fresh vegetables	Red meat	Black cohosh	Progesterone cream
Beans & legumes	Carbonated drinks	Vitex	Blue Green Algae
Orange color fruits	Caffeine	American ginseng	Seaweed
Whole grains	Alcohol	Hops	Brewer's yeast
Black licorice	Sugar	Rehmania	
Wild caught fish	All processed foods	Red clover	
Flax seeds	Dairy	Maca root	
Chia seeds		Dong quai	
Eggs			
Wheat germ			

ACNE

Foods to Eat	Foods to Avoid	Herbs	Nutritional Support
Flaxseed oil	Processed foods	Acidophilus	Zrii
Hemp seed/oil	Fried foods	Burdock root	Radiance C
Chia seed/oil	Sugar	Dandelion leaves	Vita-Synergy
Garlic	Dairy	Milk thistle	Barley Greens
Almonds	Wheat		Just Carrots
Beets	Chocolate		Colloidal silver
Grapes	Alcohol		Probiotic
Strawberries	Corn		
Pineapple	Soda		
Organic fruits	Coffee		
Dark leafy greens	Black tea		
Organic vegetables			
Cabbage			

Note: Following proper food combining rules and doing a cleanse will resolve acne when you apply the above guidelines.

INSOMNIA

Foods to Eat	Foods to Avoid	Herbs	Nutritional Support
Leafy greens	Coffee	Hydroxytryptophan	Ocean Minerals
Sunflower seeds	Black tea	Melatonin	Innate Bone Response
Brewer's yeast	Chocolate	Passion flower	D-Stress Plus
Turkey (organic)	Alcohol	Valerian	Sleep Aid
Tuna fish	Sugar	Hops	Zrii
Kefir	Sweet fruits	Chamomile	
Brown rice			
Raw organic almonds			
Raw walnuts			
Steel cut oats			

Consume Healing Foods--Avoid Deceptive Foods

SINUSITIS

Foods to Eat	Foods to Avoid	Herbs	Nutritional Support
Horseradish	Coffee	Garlic	Acerola Powder
Onions	Black tea	Ginger	Vitamin C
Egg yolk	Chocolate	Peppermint	Vitamin A
Pumpkin	Alcohol	Spearmint	
Carrot	Sugar		
Leafy vegetables	Sweet fruits		
Tomato	Breads		
Mango	Fermented foods		
Papaya	Salt		
	Fried foods		
Juices:			
Fresh citrus juice			
Vegetable juices			

NOTE: In a netty pot (which irrigates sinuses) add 1 tsp. salt (not iodized), 1 tsp. baking soda, 1 tsp. xylitol, and 3 drops tea tree oil, and pour in warm water. Irrigate the sinuses 1-2 times a day. Get plenty of fresh air and open up your living area windows to bring in clean air.

COLITIS

Foods to Eat	Foods to Avoid	Herbs	Nutritional Support
Wheat grass	Fruit	Boswellia	Lactobacillus
Ground flax seed	Fruit juices	Plantain leaf Marshmal-	Acidophilus
Cooked yams	Spicy foods	low root Yellow dock	Grapefruit seed
Bananas	Dairy	root	extract
Blended vegetables	Fried foods	Chamomile	
Raw vegetable juices,		Peppermint	
especially carrot		Licorice	
Oatmeal			
Raw honey			
Crushed garlic w/ honey			
Cold spinach soup			

IN ADDITION: Make a congee tea of various herbs listed above.

DIABETES

Foods to Eat	Foods to Avoid	Herbs	Nutritional Support
Grapefruit	All flour	Bittermelon	Magnesium
Dark leafy greens	White rice	Fenugreek	Chromium
Oatmeal	Sugar	Ceylon "true"	Alpha-Lipoic Acid
Raw vegetables	Glucose	cinnamon	Coenzyme Q10
Legumes	Dextrose	Amla-Indian Goose-	Omega-3 fatty acids
Sprouts	MSG	berry	Chia seeds
Brown rice	Coffee	Tulsi leaves	
Whole grains	Black tea	Gymnema Sylvestre	
Raw almonds & cashews	Chocolate		
Celery	Alcohol		
Cucumbers	Cooked potatoes		
String beans			
Onion			

NOTE: Prepare a mixture by adding equal amounts of turmeric powder and dried gooseberry powder with honey or drink equal amounts of gooseberry juice and fresh turmeric juice on an empty stomach regularly. The leaves of a mango tree also fight diabetes. Boil 3-4 fresh leaves of mango tree in the morning and drink. Add 3 tablespoons of Ceylon cinnamon to 1 liter of boiling water and simmer the mixture for 20 minutes on a low flame, then strain and drink.

DEPRESSION

Foods to Eat	Foods to Avoid	Herbs	Nutritional Support
Black licorice	Sugar	Licorice	5HTP
Apples	Caffeine	Rose petal tea	St. John's Wort
Raw cashews	Meat	Licorice tea	Coconut oil
Raw almonds	Fried foods	Sage & rosemary	Cod liver oil
Apple cider vinegar	Dairy products		Fish oil
Raw vegetables	Processed foods	*Ayurveda Herbs*	Vitamin D
Brown rice	Carbonated drinks	Brahmi	B-12
Brewer's yeast	White rice	Ashwagandha	L-Phenylalanine
	All flour products	Vacha	L-Tyrosine
Juices:	Drugs *(all)*	Mulathi	Folic acid
Onion juice		Tulsi	Niacin *(Anti-flushing)*
Dark leafy greens			
Celery, apple, cabbage			

IN ADDITION: An apple eaten with goat's milk and honey is very effective in uplifting the mood. Powder the seeds of two green cardamoms and add to one cup of boiling water, add stevia or xylitol, and drink this tea twice a day. Blend one onion with 2 cups very warm water and 4 tablespoons raw honey then drink ½ cup one to two times a day. Take yourself outside for 20 minutes of sunlight, exercise, and lots of laughter.

Almonds should be soaked in water overnight. Strain water, allow to air dry for 10 minutes, and store in the refrigerator.

CHAPTER APPLICATION:

The goal of this chapter is to inspire you and give you the tools to change your lifestyle pattern so that you will begin drinking 48 ounces of fresh vegetable juices daily and consuming 80% raw plant-based nutrients with 20% cooked plant-based nutrients. Of course, if you want to eat more raw foods, you are more than welcome to. You will want to invest in a quality juicer if you don't already have one. The recommended brands for juicers are Champion and Hurom.

THE 21-DAY PLAN:

Week One
Have your first meal of the day 80% raw, 20% cooked (or all raw if you would like; use recipes found in Chapter 7). Juice and drink 20 oz. of raw vegetable/fruit juice at the start of the day, diluting each juice with 1/3 water.

Week Two
Eat two meals following the 80/20 rule. Drink 34 oz. of raw vegetable/fruit juices, one 20 oz. juice first thing in the morning, and one 14 oz. juice between lunch and dinner. Dilute each juice with 1/3 water.

Week Three
Eat all three meals following the 80/20 rule and enjoy a "break" one day a week eating foods from your former lifestyle in moderation. Drink 48 oz. of raw vegetable/fruit juices: 20 oz. at the start of the day, then the remaining amount between meals.

You can find healing juices (top juice of choice would be Green Machine) and recipes in Chapter 7. You may juice more, as these drinks give your body live enzymes for faster recovery, and you may
eat more raw foods if you desire. Have fun experiencing the differences you will see in your skin, eyes, and energy. The more you apply, the more handsome the results.

There are so many ways in which you can heal yourself and fewer ways to get sick. In general, we as a society have become victims of our diseases instead of taking charge. You are not your disease; you may live with it, but your disease has no control over you unless you allow it. You are free to make choices and seek good counsel in order to restore what was lost. The road to quick recovery is omitting all the toxic foods and sources in your life and then introducing life-giving foods and thoughts. There is no one pill or supplement that will make your disease disappear; only through positive change, application and consistency will you start enjoying abundant life!

Choose today to do it now!

MORE RESOURCES:

ORGANIC FOODS

www.organic.org/articles/showarticle/article-206

www.living-foods.com/articles/10reasons.html

www.ota.com/news.html

www.oag.state.ny.us/environment/golf95.html

journeytoforever.org/farm_library/bobsmith.html

www.nal.usda.gov/afsic/AFSIC_pubs/srb0003.htm

www.sciencedaily.com/releases/2002/06/020603071017.htm

www.mindfully.org/Food/Organic-More-Nutritious-WorthingtonNov01.htm

www.sciencedaily.com/releases/2003/03/030304073059.htm

Comparison of Food Quality of Organically Versus Conventionally Grown Plant Foods. The Ecological Agriculture Project at MacDonald College of McGill University in Canada has published several informative reports and bibliographies on this topic.

Contact:
Ecological Agriculture Project
Box 191, MacDonald College
21,111 Lakeshore
Ste-Anne De Bellevue, Quebec
Canada H9X 1CO

GMO's

The Oiling of America by Mary G. Enig, Presented by Sally Fallon. Published by New Trends Publishing.

www.westonaprice.org/knowyourfats/canola.html

www.organicconsumers.org/supermarket/

www.slate.com/id/2193474/

www.gomestic.com/Gardening/Why-Grow-Your-Own-Vegetables.18465

Practice Food Combining and Heal Thyself

Rotting garbage does not belong in your body, so why eat it? Fermentation and digestive genocide, which increase your risk of major cellular damage, are the result of poor food combining. When fast-digesting foods get backed up behind slower digesting foods and they begin to rot, turning into toxic gases that the body somehow must release, the side-effects are numerous: gas, belching, allergies, disease, obesity and bloating. Many health practitioners have found that freedom from these issues is proper food combining.

Food combining is based on the premise that various foods are broken down and absorbed using different digestive enzymes and then metabolized in different areas of the digestive tract. For example, simple carbohydrates will ferment in the gut while the stomach is busy digesting proteins. This creates the perfect environment for disease and chronic fatigue. The solution to satisfying your weight and health goals is using the food combining technique.

You may already be eating all organic plant-based foods and still have problems. If foods are improperly combined, digestion can take up to eight hours to complete, whereas when properly combined it only takes about three hours. Save your energy for working, playing, thinking, detoxifying, and healing instead of digesting. Proper food combining also promotes a more energetic, mentally acute, emotionally stable individual who can handle stress more appropriately. Since digestion can cause oxidative damage and stress on the entire body, it would be logical to omit the garbage that forms through the process of eating. Add this technique and see the difference within one day.

> If what goes into the stomach is not properly processed in the stomach, putrification and illness will result. Most illnesses begin within the bowels and the disease is seen or felt elsewhere, giving the illusion that the foods you eat are not related to how you feel.

The general rule of food combining is that proteins and carbohydrates should never be eaten at the same time. Proteins may be eaten with non-starchy vegetables, while carbohydrates (grains, starchy vegetables) may be eaten with all vegetables as well as legumes. Fruits must be eaten alone, usually as a snack, and the same is true with dairy products. As with any rule, there are always a few exceptions. According to Patrick Donovan, N.D., of Cancer Centers of America, in Seattle, Washington, "The rational for this approach is the difference in digestion time for various food groups." Dr. Donovan explains, "Digestion is optimal if foods eaten together have roughly the same digestion time." There is no need to train your body, just your mind, as your body already knows how to digest using food combining rules.

The foundations for food combining were put into practice by Dr. William Howard Hay (1866-1940), a western medicine doctor who fell ill due to his unhealthy lifestyle. He was unsuccessful in finding a cure for himself through western medicine, so he began researching the relationship of what we eat to our physical-mental health. When Dr. Hay became very ill, he believed that the only cure was to change his pattern of eating back to a more plant-based proper food combining lifestyle. This method was and is still contrary to the conventional view of healthy eating. Dr. Hay studied all the food science that was available to him and constructed his now famous diet, "The Hay Diet," which is better known as the Food Combining Diet. He was the first person to benefit from his own improved lifestyle.

From an article entitled Why Science and Medicine Support Food Combining : "One report that strongly influenced Dr. Hay was that of Dr. Robert McCarrison, an officer in the British Army Medical Services, who observed extreme longevity in the Himalayas. The population subsisted on nuts and vegetables and fruit, mostly raw, whole grain bread, and small amounts of raw milk and cheese. He also observed that these people suffered very little disease, unlike the Europeans who imported their refined diets with them. Dr. Hay treated a lot of people with a wide range of chronic illness. He observed from his own practical experience and observation that many of these people, written off as incurable by their own doctor, recovered and then maintained good health when following his diets. By 1935 Dr. Hay was Medical Director of Hay System, Inc. and set out his ideas in 'A New Health Era'. Our own knowledge of the internal workings of the human body have progressed a long way since he wrote the book. But in harmony his observations on diet and health still remain an accurate basis for a healthy lifestyle."

When learning about proper food combining, it is important to remember that there are three cycles in which the body operates during a 24-hour period. If these cycles are ignored, ill health can be created causing the breakdown of normal system functions.

BODY CYCLES

Cycle	Time Frame	Optimal food intake
Elimination: body wastes and food debris	4:00 a.m. to 12:00 p.m.	Fruits only
Appropriation: eating and digestion	12:00 p.m. to 8:00 p.m.	Fruits if eaten before meals, vegetables with one protein or starch in proper combinations
Assimilation: absorption and usage	8:00 p.m. to 4:00 a.m.	Avoid all food during this cycle

Most people have had the experience of eating a late night meal and waking up the next morning feeling as though they had little rest. The reason for this fatigue is that during 8:00 p.m. to 4:00 a.m., the body is supposed to be absorbing nutrients and repairing the system from daily wear and tear. If digestion, a high energy activity, is occurring while the body is set for rest and healing, you will wake up the next morning feeling as if you have not received enough rest.

Food combining is still a controversial practice. Some find it ineffective and frustrating, and some have more sensitive digestive systems than others. Food combining may be less effective if you have congestion or poor absorption in the intestinal track. However, most who have tried it have found it to be the best weight reduction method, and others feel more clarity and energy. There is no harm caused by the food combining lifestyle, only enhanced health. Experiment for yourself—try it for the next 21 days and experience the difference. Listen to your body, as some are more sensitive, while others have hearty digestive tracts. What works for one person may not fully work for another person. Since you have applied Chapter 4 to your lifestyle already, eating 80 percent raw and 20 percent cooked food, this should be an easy and complementary addition to the practice of eating Food Beautiful.

If you're still not convinced, here are some of the effects of improperly combining your food:

ILL EFFECTS OF IMPROPER FOOD COMBINING:

- Excess energy expenditure by the body, leading to fatigue.
- Enzyme depletion, leading to aging and disease.
- Increased tissue toxins and a decreased ability for the body to eliminate toxins, leading to a host of problems.

- Putrification of foods in the intestines leading to increased gas, bloating, and poor elimination from the bowels. Putrification robs the body of vital nutrients to create healthy, life-giving cells free of disease and illness.
- Fermentation of starches, sugars, and protein, leading to the production of unusable substances like carbon dioxide and acetic acid, which act like poisonous gases in the body.

All these factors combined may lead to impaired body function and ill health. To derive sustenance from foods they must be properly digested. Anything that reduces the digestive power favors bacterial activity. Therefore, overeating, eating right before a work out, eating when cold or hot, eating when feverish, eating when in pain, eating when not hungry, eating when worried/anxious/fearful/angry—all of these can lead to increased bacterial activity. Try to spend 10-20 minutes before a meal diffusing any negative or stressful emotions or thoughts by relaxing to easy listening music and doing deep breathing combined with stretching. Taking the time now to learn and practice the basic rules of food combining is guaranteed to make a huge difference in how you feel.

RULES FOR PROPER FOOD COMBINING:

- Protein and vegetables combine perfectly! Do not mix starches with protein.
- Starches and vegetables combine perfectly! Do not mix starches with protein.
- Fruit must be eaten alone. Start the day with fruit and avoid eating it between meals (apples are an exception).
- Do not eat any melon with other fruits.
- Since juicing fruits and vegetables extracts the fibers, they combine well when freshly juiced.
- Avoid eating meat. Occasional consumption of organic meat can be healing and is best digested with non-starchy vegetables.
- Protein then starches: For optimal digestion when eating throughout the day, have your protein at lunch and starch at dinner, as the protein is digested in the lower end of the stomach while the starch is digested in the upper part of the stomach.
- Do not eat fats and proteins together in a meal unless you are having a salad or significant amount of fresh vegetables. The fat has a distinct inhibiting influence on the secretion of gastric juices that are required for protein digestion.
- Do not mix sugars with protein! The sugars inhibit the gastric juices needed to digest protein. Sugars need to be digested in the intestines, or else they end up fermenting in the stomach. Take sugars alone or with vegetables only, so they pass through the stomach quickly.
- Dairy (which counts as a fat) should be eaten alone or with fresh raw vegetables or semi-sweet fruits (like mango, papaya, and avocado). Here a couple of examples of combinations that digest well together: smoothies with kefir, kale, and frozen mango; a salad with raw goat cheese and beans.

- When eating an abundance of vegetables, you can usually get away with having fat, a little bit of sugar, and meat in one meal. For example, you can have vegetables with raspberry vinaigrette (which has sugar in it) with some fish and flax seed oil on top.
- More than one kind of starch at a meal can lead to overeating, which leads to bacterial activity.
- Be sure to drink water 15-20 minutes before meals as water with a starchy meal weakens the action of the saliva on the starch.
- Chew your starches and all foods very well (30-50 chews) before swallowing.
- If you eat a dessert, follow it up with a green salad to push the food through.

EXCEPTIONS

- You can have fats and proteins in the same meal only if you have an abundance of green, un cooked vegetables.
- You can have an apple with any meal or at any time of the day as it has a neutral effect on the stomach and helps to satiate hunger, balance blood sugar, and reduce fermentation in the colon and small intestines.
- Salad dressings that have sugars in them are fine on salads, as the green vegetables help to carry them through to the intestines.
- Celery, all varieties of lettuce and dark leafy greens (kale, collards and spinach) combine well with any fruit, or after any meal. If you have a salad with fruit, leave out all other vegetables.
- Eggs combine well with other proteins, fats, or dairy, but not with starches. However, egg whites are neutral and combine well with almost any food.
- Freshly juiced fruits and vegetables combine well.
- Acidic fruits such as grapefruit, lemons, and tangerines mix well with nuts, as the acids of the stomach do not delay the digestion of nuts. For example, a good combination breakfast meal would be a grapefruit, orange, apple, or pineapple, with nuts and some avocado. However, I would again suggest having this at the beginning of the day. Some people may still find this to slightly impair digestion. If so, then avoid having nuts with acid fruit.
- Even though tomatoes are a fruit they can be combined with meat only when eating lots of leafy greens. Tomatoes eaten with meat or starches is not a good combination.
- Though starches are not good to combine with protein, brown rice with beans or fish combines fairly well together.
- Avocados are a fruit and a fat so they combine well with both fruits and fats.

Note: Food Beautiful recommends avoiding all meat as it is acidic, dead, low in nutrients, and filled with antibiotics (if not organic) and hormones. Occasionally eating organic meat can be medicinal for those with weak constitutions. It is not recommended to eat meat more than one time a week, and even more preferred to have it only once a month, if necessary. It is best to avoid the use of all meats if you are suffering from cancer, or digestive, hormone or tumor related ailments. Digesting meat overworks your pancreas and digestive enzymes and pulls calcium out of your muscles, tendons, and ligaments to neutralize its acidic constitution. In addition, the breakdown of meat in the body requires oxygen, leading to a process called oxidation, which produces free radicals. And you probably already know that free radicals cause premature aging. Modern science, by the preponderance of evidence, believes 80 percent or more of the damage done to the body is the result of free radicals. The more difficult the digestion, such as in digesting meat, the more oxidation is required to break down foods. Having too many free radicals is not healing, but destructive to the body.

A superior replacement for meat is food with amino acids, as these are the foundation of what we call protein. All plant-based foods have amino acids that create the proteins your body needs. For meat lovers it will be satisfying to consume moderate amounts of organic raw goat's milk or kefir, avocados, sprouts, mushrooms, and nuts and seeds with fresh vegetables. Raw goat's milk has the protein structure closest to a human mother's milk and is pre-digested with high quality amino acids and probiotics. It is much easier to digest than meat, requiring less time to break down the molecules.

Proper Food Combining Examples

Time	Meal	Food
Upon Arising	Snack	2 pieces of fruit, or 16 oz. vegetable-fruit juice
20 min. after arising	Breakfast	• Oatmeal, coconut milk, chia seeds, xylitol • Cinnamon toast: Coconut oil spread over toasted sprouted grain bread topped with xylitol and cinnamon • Smoothie: Frozen fruit, coconut kefir, and kale • More ideas in Chapter 7
Mid-Morning	Snack	Green tea, veggie juice
12:00-2:00 p.m.	Lunch	• Salad with spinach, romaine, feta cheese, beans and olive oil-based dressing • Veggie wrap with hummus, sprouts, black beans, brown rice, and shredded veggies

Proper Food Combining Examples

Time	Meal	Food
2:00-4:00 p.m.	Snack	• An apple with 2 tablespoons raw almond butter • Baby carrots or celery with hummus • Vegetable juice (recipes in <u>Chapter 7</u>) • Celery sticks with salsa or raw nuts • One cup coconut or goat kefir with chopped apples, cinnamon, nutmeg and stevia • Organic raw food bars. For quick fixes you can get health food bars that do not follow the food combining rules, since these are only eaten once a day or less. Some good bars that are raw or minimally processed are: Lara Bar™, Organic Food Bar™, Bobo's™ Oatmeal bars. • 10-12 raw almonds, which can help balance blood sugar. To make them even more absorbable, soak the raw nuts in water overnight, drain, rinse, and dry for 1 hour. Store in fridge.
5:00-7:00 p.m.	Dinner	• Veggies stir fried in coconut oil and raw soy sauce (with spices) and wild caught salmon • Sprouted grain pasta with organic tomato sauce and grated almond parmesan cheese • Look for more recipes in **Chapter 7**! *Note: Do not eat later than 8:00 p.m.*

CHAPTER 5 APPLICATION:

Take the next 21 days to fully implement proper food combining.
(Note: Do this six days a week and enjoy one day off.)

Week one: Properly combine breakfast.
Week two: Properly combine breakfast and lunch.
Week three: Properly combine all three meals.

Follow this star guide rating in Chapter 7 for levels of combination. You will also find the rating key in the beginning part of the recipe section and next to each recipe.

★★★★ Perfect Food Combining (100%)
★★★ Good Food Combining (75%)
★★ Half Food Combining (50%)
★ Not Following Food Combining (Less than 50%)

OTHER GUIDELINES & SUGGESTIONS:

- The recipes in Chapter 7 each have a star rating so you can follow the food combining rules with better success. If you have a serious disease or illness, it is in your best interest to follow the food combining rules 90-100% of the time.
- Great juice combination: ½ cucumber, 3 celery sticks, 3 leaves of kale, ½ apple, 2 carrots, ¼ purple cabbage, handful parsley. Add ginger, turmeric, and/or cayenne for extra nutrition. See more juicing tips and recipes in chapter 7.
- Refined foods are to be avoided. Stick to foods that look like they came out of the earth. The occasional splurge on junk food can be done one time a week, but be careful not to overeat.
- Continue to speak words of truth over yourself. Examples: "I have full freedom from _____", "I take up the action of _____ (persistence, self control, faith, pushing through moments of vulnerability)", and "My body is in full submission to my heart's desires." With faith and action the Creator will give you your heart's desires! Remember, your mental pictures and actions become your reality, so start seeing and feeling the difference.

TRAVEL TIPS:

When you are traveling or eating out, it is a health saver to have with you what we call a "Food Beautiful Travel Kit". This kit allows you the ability to create Food Beautiful options when you are not in your own home or kitchen. This little kit will help you avoid unhealthy sauces, spices, dressings, sugars, salt and dips by enabling you to design your own creative combinations for jazzing up foods.

Never leave home without this handy tool. You can carry it in your purse, brief case, or any bag you like to travel with. You can even get all you-can-drink free lemonade while eating out (find out how on the next page).

ITEMS NEEDED TO MAKE YOUR OWN FOOD BEAUTIFUL TRAVEL KIT:

- A clear 4x6 inch or larger vinyl travel bag
- Seven 2-3 ounce containers (such as pyrex or tupperware) filled with:
  - Sea salt
  - Xylitol and/or stevia (sugar replacement)
  - Ready-mixed spices (see below)
  - Bragg Liquid Aminos™ (soy sauce and salad dressing replacement that mixes well with olive oil)
  - Extra virgin olive oil
  - Organic tea of choice like peppermint, chamomile, or green tea
  - Chia seeds (whole or ground) - Chia is a healthy way to get fiber, EFA's, vitamins, and minerals (learn more about chia in Chapter 4). Add 1 tablespoon chia seeds to 1-2 cups of water or fresh juice and stir until mixed together. Drink within 5-10 minutes. This is a great nutrient-packed food that curbs appetite and reduces bad food cravings.
- Travel fork-spoon
- Travel can opener

QUICK RECIPE FOR READY-MIXED SPICES:

1/8 tsp. white pepper
1 tsp. garlic powder
1 tsp. dill or basil
1/8 tsp. cayenne pepper
1 tsp. sea salt
1/10 tsp. stevia powder (optional)
1 Tbsp. of granular onion powder

SOME GOOD IDEAS WHILE EATING OUT:

- Make your own healthy lemonade (for free!): Ask for 4 fresh lemon slices, then squeeze them into your water and add stevia or xylitol.
- Ask for brown rice instead of white, extra veggies, and dressing on the side. Use your Bragg Liquid Aminos, olive oil, spices, and a fresh lemon.
- Avoid creamy soups and pick vegetable-based soups.
- Make healthy iced tea: Ask for 1 cup of hot water and 1 cup of ice. Place tea bag from travel kit in hot water, add xylitol or stevia, steep, and then pour over ice.
- Ask for an open-faced sandwich with an extra side of lightly steamed veggies, and use your Bragg Liquid Aminos and olive oil to dress up the veggies.

- Ask for a cup of salsa, sample cup of soup, side of mustard, side of relish, side of guacamole, side of tomato sauce used for pastas, soy sauce, or ½ cup of plain yogurt (better option) to jazz up any side dish or salad.

Use these ideas to create a variety of different flavors to make salads or veggies tasty. Get creative and don't be afraid to ask! By properly combining foods and following Food Beautiful principles, you will be amazed at how delicious food can be!

FOOD COMBINING CHART

Note: Food Beautiful does not recommend eating meat or animal based products. However they are included in this chart so that if you do eat these you know how to combine them properly. Some of the foods below naturally fit into multiple categories. Exceptions to the rules are listed IF you are eating the Food Beautiful Diet.

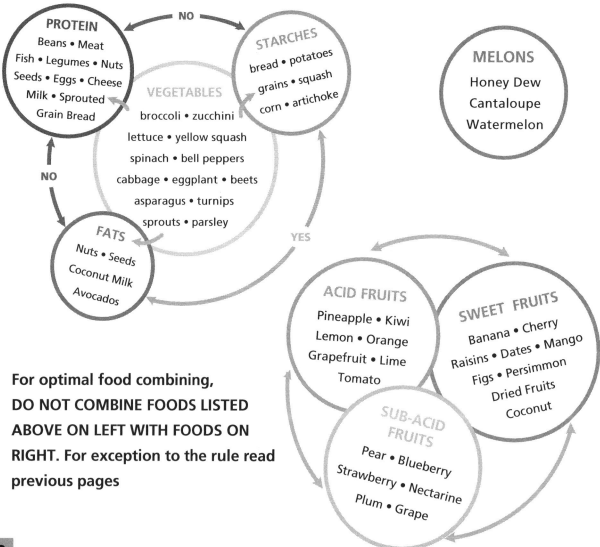

PROTEIN
Beans • Meat
Fish • Legumes • Nuts
Seeds • Eggs • Cheese
Milk • Sprouted
Grain Bread

STARCHES
bread • potatoes
grains • squash
corn • artichoke

MELONS
Honey Dew
Cantaloupe
Watermelon

VEGETABLES
broccoli • zucchini
lettuce • yellow squash
spinach • bell peppers
cabbage • eggplant • beets
asparagus • turnips
sprouts • parsley

FATS
Nuts • Seeds
Coconut Milk
Avocados

ACID FRUITS
Pineapple • Kiwi
Lemon • Orange
Grapefruit • Lime
Tomato

SWEET FRUITS
Banana • Cherry
Raisins • Dates • Mango
Figs • Persimmon
Dried Fruits
Coconut

SUB-ACID FRUITS
Pear • Blueberry
Strawberry • Nectarine
Plum • Grape

For optimal food combining, DO NOT COMBINE FOODS LISTED ABOVE ON LEFT WITH FOODS ON RIGHT. For exception to the rule read previous pages

Exercise and Breathe With Intention

Oxygen is universally necessary for the existence of all living things. Oxygen is extracted from the air we breathe and brought into our lungs, passing through the blood vessels that surround our lungs. With every exchange of breath, inhale and exhale, we take in oxygen and release carbon dioxide and toxins stored in our tissues and blood. Seventy percent of all the toxins produced in our bodies are removed through breathing.

Deep breathing and aerobic exercise will increase oxygen utilization in the blood while releasing toxins stored in fat cells and various organs. The tri-fold combination of deep breathing, physical exercise, and perspiration opens the pores and allows the body to release undesirable toxins. If you are not breathing deeply enough or getting enough exercise, you may have a build up of toxins in your organs and tissues. Thankfully, bad habits can be broken, and reverse-deep breathing techniques and dynamic exercise can rebuild healthy new cells.

> Seventy percent of all the toxins produced in our bodies are removed through breathing

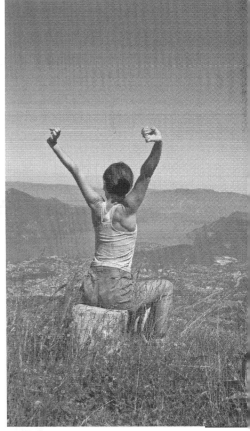

All doctors and scientists agree: "Every cell in the body requires oxygen to function properly. The brain alone uses at least 12% of the total oxygen that people inhale."[1] Oxygen passes quickly from the alveoli in the lungs directly through the air-blood barrier into your blood. Carbon dioxide moves from the blood to the alveoli and is exhaled. The International Breath Institute in Colorado has found that 70% of your body's natural toxins are released during exhalation and inefficient exhalation is the primary cause of hypoxia, which simply means that there is an insufficient supply of oxygen to the cells in the brain and other important parts of the body.[2] Shallow chest breathing gives rise to oxygen deficiencies as there are very few blood vessels surrounding the upper lobes of the lungs. Most of your blood vessels surround the lower lobes of the lung. Deep abdominal breathing sustains optimum oxygen levels while having good mechanics.[3] During exercise, it is possible to breathe in and out more than 100 liters of air per minute and extract three liters of oxygen from this air per minute,[4] which is exactly why regular exercise is one of the best things you can do to help prevent illness, preserve health and longevity, and enhance quality of life.

Apart from breathing, the next best way to detox is through your skin. Your body is constantly excreting toxins from your internal and external environment. The lungs excrete toxic gases from the blood and absorb fresh oxygen through the air. Deep breathing and exhalation actively release toxins from the environment, mind, and body while simultaneously improving your physical beauty, mental clarity, and mood, which is essential for weight loss and disease prevention. Scientists at the University of Stirling in Scotland discovered that as cellular toxin levels rise, the thyroid, adrenals, and other weight-regulating glands become sluggish. In an attempt to protect these vital organs, the body forms additional fat as storage for these toxins. Thankfully, up to 70% of toxins are easily converted into gases that are expelled through deep breaths. Proper breathing can dramatically lessen one's toxic load, leaving more room in the cells for an optimal exchange of oxygen.

We all know that the more you move your body with intention, the more weight you shed. If you feel sick and tired you must give energy to get it! Your body is designed to move and work at various intensity levels. Exercise increases the body's level of endorphins, chemicals in the brain that reduce pain and induce a sense of well-being. Thus, exercise appears to help improve mood and energy levels and may even help relieve depression.[5] Exercise should be done 3-4 times a week in conjunction with your lifestyle diet of fresh herbs, fresh juices, and regular total body detox as discussed in earlier chapters. The better you start to feel, the more action you take; it's a self-perpetuating cycle! At any moment you can start a new life with a shift in your thoughts and actions. Don't let your past keep you from your future.

Your body was created to adapt to the environment and the stress under which it is placed. Participating in dynamic exercise will increase your health, leanness and joy in various stages. Each time you reach a level that feels comfortable back off for one week then increase your intensity so your body does not adapt. It is important to increase the intensity and duration of your exercise, pushing through each uncomfortable stage until you reach your desired health, beauty, and weight goals.

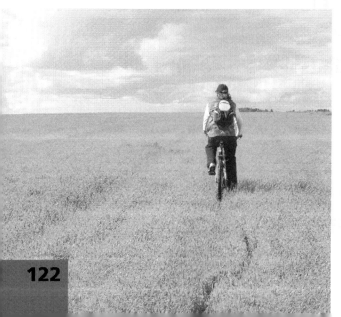

key to exercising is to make sure you are doing it tively. There are three important variables: length time, frequency (times you workout per week), and tensity (workload). Your exercise program should two stages; six weeks of building in which you ally increase workout time, frequency and intensity, lowed by a seventh week for recovery at half the out intensity, time, and frequency. Then start the all over again. Keep cycling the building periods six weeks with every seventh week at half the time, quency, and intensity. For beginners, or those who have not been working out regularly, start with 15 minutes of aerobic exercise four days a week such as running, walking, using an elliptical machine or treadmill, doing aerobics, cycling or any other activity that makes your heart beat faster. Each week add five minutes to your workout until you have reached your desired time of 45 minutes or more of exercise. As a rule of thumb never dramatically bump up your exercise time, as this could lead to injury or discouragement.

To better understand the appropriate intensity level for your body, consider the "talk test" measure. You want to exercise hard enough to have a difficult time carrying on a conversation. Once you reach that level back off slightly. You can use the formula below to exercise at your optimum training level. Use the following intervals in any combination with exercise types like walking, jogging, running, aerobics, and dance workouts. It is most effective to have two workouts at the "talk test" level and two workouts above the "talk test" level per week. Again, if you are just starting to exercise, start with 15 minutes and gradually build up time and intensity over six weeks.

Here is a simple equation that accurately measures your fitness level and intensity zone for workouts, using the following:

Maximum Heart Rate (MHR) = 220 - Your Age.

Fat-burning Zone (FUR) = 55 to 75% MHR

Performance Enhancement Rate (PER) = 75 - 85% MHR

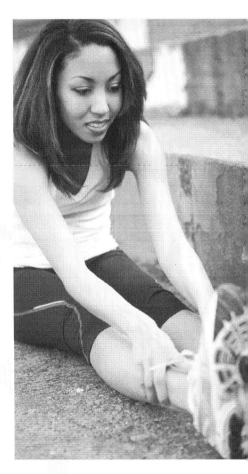

Use this equation to calculate your Maximum Heart Rate so you can find your different workout zones, as listed above:

MHR: 220 – Your Age = _____ BPM (Beats Per Minute)

Your heart should not exceed the number of beats per minute of your Maximum Heart Rate (MHR) during exercise. The safe zone for exercise is the Fat-burning Zone (FUR) which is 55 to 75% MHR. Most people should shoot for two workouts a week in the 55% MHR Zone with higher intensity workouts at the 75% MHR Zone. For experienced athletes, make your high intensity days at the Performance Enhancement Rate (PER) which is 75 to 85% MHR.

Example of how to calculate the Zone Heart Rates for a 40-year-old person:

MHR: 220 - 40 = 180 BPM

FUR: 55 – 75% of 180 = 99 to 135 BPM

PER: 75 – 85% of 180 = 135 to 153 BPM

INTERVAL TRAINING FOR ALL TYPES

For the already active adult, begin adding interval workouts two times a week to your schedule of four or more workouts per week. Interval workouts have a short period of high intensity followed by a recovery period of lower intensity. This produces a thermogenic response in the body that continues to burn fat for as long as six to eight hours afterwards. You can vary the length of the higher intensity portion. The more in shape you get, the more time you'll want for interval training!

Beginner Level Intervals
5 min. easy warm up 12 min. of repeating 1 min. above "talk test" then 2 min. at "talk test" level 5 min. cool down
Intermediate Level Intervals
7-10 min. easy warm up 20-25 min. of repeating 1 min. above "talk test" level then 1:30 min. at "talk test" level 7-10 min. cool down
Advanced Level Intervals
10 min. warm up 25-35 min. of repeating 1 min. above "talk test" level then 1 min. at "talk test" level 10 min. cool down
Personalize Your Workout Routine
1. Calculate MHR, FUR, and PER zones. 2. Pick an exercise. 3. Start the workout with 5-10 minutes of warm-up. 4. After the warm-up, increase the speed, tension or incline so you can reach desired zone. 5. End the workout with 5-10 minutes of cool down. 6. Track your workouts by recording time, speed, and intensity.

DIAPHORETIC HERBS THAT INDUCE PERSPIRATION

Angelica	**Camphor**	**Garlic**	**Rosemary**
Basil	**Catnip**	**Ginger**	**Sassafras**
Blessed Thistle	**Cayenne**	**Hyssop**	**Yarrow**
Butcher's Broom	**Chamomile**	**Lavender**	
Calendula	**Elecampane**	**Oregano**	

As you exercise, especially at the higher intensities, you should be sweating. If you need some help in this area, diaphoretic herbs may help. They induce perspiration and are highly beneficial for detoxification, fevers, and colds. You can make teas using loose-leaf herbs or buy encapsulated formulas. If you make tea I would follow the recommendations on the containers, as each herb varies. Drink these teas 2 times a day between meals.

BREATHING EXERCISE

Simple Breathing Exercise

Do this lying down initially since those who are unused to efficient breathing may feel slight dizziness. Place a book or some lightweight object on the abdomen. Inhale to a count of four and exhale to a count of six. This is one round. Only do up to ten rounds initially. Slowly increase up to 30 rounds over a few weeks. Then double the exhalation, so you inhale to a count of four and exhale to a count of eight. This depends on individual capacity, so take extreme care not to exert. If you feel breathless or dizzy, you are exerting, and must learn to do lesser counts and lesser rounds till your lungs can accommodate this new skill.[6]

Reverse Breathing Exercise

Below is an excerpt taken from **http://internalart.tripod.com/the%20art%20of%20meditation/breathing.htm**

Check out the YouTube Video called Reverse Breathing–Mingmen/Dantian to see how this is done.

The stomach contracts as we breathe in, and expands as we breathe out. This technique is the reverse of the normal breathing. It helps to clean our internal system through effective circulation of oxygen while removing the free radicals from the body. During the time that you exhale let out negative thoughts or emotions and when you inhale breath in positive actions and thoughts. Be very cautious when practicing Reverse Breathing. Do not practice more than three minutes at a time, and don't force it or you may injure yourself. Please take the time to visit the websites listed on this site, so you are clear on the mechanics of reverse breathing as it is more difficult to practice than Normal Breathing.

- Stand or sit with feet shoulder width apart and hands relaxed to your sides or resting on your legs. Loosen any tight clothing and close your eyes. Quietly observe your breath, removing all busy and negative thoughts. Before starting have your tongue lightly touching the upper roof of the mouth, and tuck in your chin. Tilt up your pelvis correctly. And now you are ready to begin with the reverse breathing part. Start with exhaling.

- Exhaling: the thoracic diaphragm moves upward, while the pelvic diaphragm moves downward. At the same time, the stomach expands on all four sides, creating a vacuum effect in the center. Your belly should comfortably bulge out while exhaling.

- Inhaling: the belly contracts from all four sides. While the thoracic diaphragm moves downward, the pelvic diaphragm is moving upward. Your stomach should feel like you are sucking it in. If you need to, place your hands on your belly so you can better perform this breathing technique.

- Do this continuously for 2-3 minutes (30-50 full breathing cycles) in a slow, relaxed manner, only exhaling consciously through your nose. Then relax for 30 sec. and resume the exercise. As time progresses, increase practice time of reverse breathing to 5-6 minutes.[7]

FOUR STEPS TO BETTER OXYGENATION

The steps are listed in optimal order for effective oxygen increase:

1. Practice Deep Energy Breathing: Sit up straight and take 20 to 30 quick, panting breaths. Only your belly should move, not your chest. Then take a deep breath and hold it for 20-30 seconds. Exhale completely by pressing your hand against your belly. This puts pressure on your lungs, forcing out more of the used air.

2. Exercise: Three times a week, complete 40-60 minutes of aerobic exercise and 20-30 minutes of strength training.

3. Eat oxygen rich foods: Juice and eat alkalinizing foods that quickly deliver living enzymes, minerals, and vitamins for smooth blood flow and oxygen saturation. Examples: sprouts, fruits and vegetables (especially dark leafy greens, beets, berries, mangos, fresh figs, grapes, broccoli, onions, lemons, tomatoes), garlic, chia seeds, quinoa and seeds.

4. Practice good posture and maintain good spinal alignment.[8]

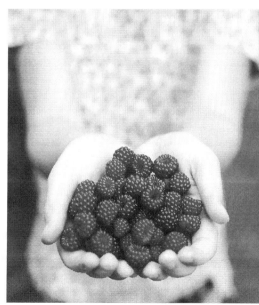

CHAPTER 6 APPLICATION:

Over the next six weeks begin doing 3-4 workouts and gradually increase the time and intensity. Your exercise program should have a building stage of six weeks followed by a back-off period in the seventh week at half the time, frequency, and intensity. Never go above your maximum heart rate zone unless you are experienced. Use the Fat Burning Zones to tailor the intensity of your workouts. Beginners should stay in the FUR zone and more experienced adults can use the PER zone for higher intensity workouts.

Encourage perspiration with diaphoretic herbs. Add breathing exercises 2-3 times a day - before and after your workouts, as well as at various times throughout the day. Once you start getting in shape, feeling renewed energy, and experiencing the joy of a strong body, you will never go back!

1   Hamner, Daniel. "The Oxygen Cure." Accessed Jan. 8, 2010, http://www.activeforever.com/t-oxygen-cure.aspx

2   Akthar, Shameem. "Waiting to Exhale." June 23, 2008; accessed Jan. 8, 2010, http://www.lifepositive.com

3   "The Importance of Oxygen." April 7, 2009; accessed Jan. 8, 2010, http://pharmacyworld.org/2009/04/the-importance-of-oxygen/

4   Brain, Joseph D. "Exchanging Oxygen and Carbon Dioxide." August 2006; accessed Jan. 8, 2010, http://www.merck.com/mmhe/sec04/ch038/ch038d.html?qt=exchanging%20oxygen%20and %20carbon%20dioxide&alt=sh

5   Johnston, Brian D. "Benefits of Exercise." Online Merck Manual. September 2007.

6   Ibid

7   http://internalart.tripod.com/the%20art%20of%20meditation/breathing.htm

8   http://www.activeforever.com

CHAPTER 7

Eat Delicious *Food Beautiful* Recipes and Juices

Food is your friend! When you use food correctly, the health results are astounding. Now that you have learned all the principles of Food Beautiful, it is time to start practicing the actions of combining, cooking, and eating simply marvelous foods. To become 'beautifully healthy' you need to eat the Food Beautiful way; eating this way will help you find freedom from illness as a result of this process. To make the method simple, I have laid out some guiding principles.

HERE ARE THE FOODS YOU SHOULD EAT:

Raw... Raw... Veggies & Fruits!

Eat as many raw vegetables as you would like. The more color you have in your diet the larger spectrum of nutrients you will obtain. Eat 2-3 pieces of fresh fruits a day; however, if you eat dried fruits limit the intake to one or two times a week and eat no more than one handful at a time. If you have candida, cancer, diabetes, or low blood sugar you should avoid dried fruits all together. My favorite fruits and the ones I recommend are: papaya, grapefruit, apples, berries, ripe bananas, and fresh figs.

Plant foods packed with proteins

The following are all wonderful sources of protein: sprouts, seeds (chia, flax, sesame, sunflower, pumpkin, etc.), avocados, beans & legumes, grains such as quinoa, vegetables, and nuts. Have no more than 1/8 cup of nuts at a time so that you do not overtax the liver. If you have had your gallbladder removed you should always take a digestive enzyme or avoid nuts all together. Nuts and seeds digest easier in the presence of dark leafy greens.

Whole grains

Grains supply you with ample phytonutrients, but should not be overused. It is ideal to choose from grains that are closest to their original state because whole grains slow down the digestion and do

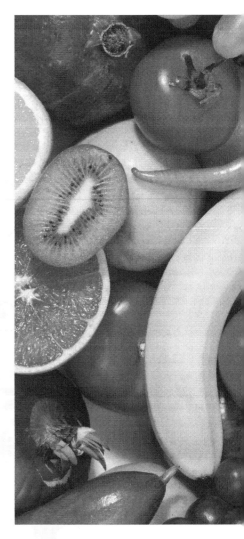

The more color you have in your diet the larger spectrum of nutrients you will obtain.

not spike your blood sugar levels. My favorites are sprouted grains (breads, tortillas, and bagels), or whole cooked grains (brown rice, oat groats, steel cut oats, millet, buckwheat, quinoa, spelt, and kamut). Watch out for misleading packaging that says 100% whole grain, or gluten-free, which means it is from a whole grain, but is likely to be refined and may contain added sugars. Gluten-free breads are not necessarily low in sugar or good for you; they are just free of gluten, and could contain high amounts of added fruit sweeteners. If you buy bread it is best to buy sprouted grain bread or whole spelt grain bread. If you sprout a glutinous grain, like wheat, it disables the gluten in it by transforming it into an amino acid.

Eat mostly vegan, but don't be vegan.

I believe that humans thrive by eating plant-based foods because they are packed with enzymes, vitamins, minerals, and fibers. In the past, most ancient cultures ate animal meat and dairy—occasionally. However, since we have combined technology and food production, 50-70% of people's diets now consist of animal-based foods. A sick person who has eaten meat all of his (or her) life is not deficient in animal meat; he is deficient in living enzymes, vitamins, and minerals that have been drawn out of the body. It takes a great deal of effort to break down the muscles of another animal and more effort and expense for you to recover from eating it. I am not saying you should never eat meat; I am saying to be mindful and aware of the ramifications to your health from eating animal-based foods. The strongest animals like bears, elephants, and buffalo eat only plants. For someone who has been eating meat 1-2 times a day, begin by reducing your meat by half. Ideally, you should eat wild caught fish or organic free range meat 1-2 times a month, not 1-2 times a day. I eat plant-based foods 95% of the time and eat meat once a month and eggs once a week. Don't be a snob about your food and lose friends over it, just make them aware of your choices and hopefully they will respect your choice to be healthy.

Dairy from goats

I never recommend eating dairy from a cow; the protein molecule is too large for us to properly digest. I do recommend that underweight, frail, or highly active children and adults should eat small amounts of goat yogurt or kefir every other day. Also, coconut milk and coconut kefir is just as healthy as and cheaper than goat dairy. Be wary of imitation cheeses; if they are not vegan, they contain a cow milk protein called casein, which is cancer-forming. Read labels carefully!

Healthy sweeteners

Use stevia, xylitol, and agave nectar as your main source(s) of sweetener. You can use raw honey and maple syrup in small amounts. Use xylitol in equal parts to other sweeteners in recipes, such as honey or maple syrup. Agave nectar is a one to one replacement for honey. One half tsp powdered stevia is equivalent to one fourth cup sugar.

Use this key for choosing recipes that follow the Food Combining rules:
(Refer to Chapter 5 for learning the basics of Food Combining)

★★★★ Perfect Food Combining (100%)
★★★ Good Food Combining (75%)
★★ Half Food Combining (50%)
★ Not Following Food Combining (Less than 50%)

BREAKFAST

Nut or Seed Milk ★★★★

Ingredients:

1 cup organic raw almonds
  (or any other seed or nut)
3 cups purified water
1 tsp lemon juice

1 tsp vanilla extract
⅛ tsp sea salt
¼ cup maple syrup or pitted dates (optional)

Tools:

Unbleached cheesecloth
Blender or food processor

Preparations:

Place the 1 cup of organic raw almonds in a medium size bowl and soak them in water overnight. Note: It won't hurt the almonds if you soak them longer than 12 hours. The next day, discard the old water and place the almonds and 3 cups of fresh water into the blender and blend for 30 seconds. Strain the liquid through cheesecloth to remove the large pieces, and then return the liquid to the blender. Add the lemon juice, maple syrup or dates, vanilla, and sea salt and process again.

Place into a glass jar to preserve the taste and freshness. Can be stored in the fridge for up to 3-4 days.

Date-Pecan Squares ✶✶

Ingredients:

1 cup pitted dates	1 cup raisins
½ cup pecans	2 cups unsweetened shredded coconut
1 tsp vanilla extract	

Preparations:

In a food processor grind pecans into a fine meal. Add dates and raisins and process until a dough-like consistency is reached. By hand, work in ½ cup of the coconut. Sprinkle ¾ cup of the coconut in a small cookie pan with sides or square baking dish. Spread the date pecan mixture evenly in the pan. Top with the remaining coconut.

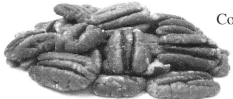

Cover and refrigerate. When chilled, cut into squares and serve. Makes 8 squares.

Date Coconut Logs ✶✶✶

Ingredients:

2 cups pitted dates
1 cup unsweetened shredded coconut
½ cup apple juice

Preparations:

In a food processor using the "S" blade, or in a blender, grind the dates and apple juice until a dough-like consistency is reached.

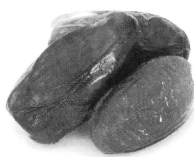

With wet hands shape the dough into logs. Roll each log in coconut until coated. Serves 5.

Raw Oatmeal ★★★★

Note: Unrefined whole grains provide essential amino acids and B vitamins to help with stress. If you do not want to use coconut milk, add another ½ cup water to the recipe.

Ingredients:

½-¾ cup steel cut oats	¾ cups water
¼ tsp cinnamon	2 TBSP unsweetened shredded
1 TBSP wheat germ	coconut (optional)
2 pinches nutmeg	1 apple, chopped
5-10 drops liquid stevia (or to taste)	1 TBSP ground chia seed

Preparations:

In a large bowl, cover, steel cut oats, cinnamon, wheat germ, nutmeg, coconut flakes, stevia, coconut milk, and water. Soak overnight at room temperature or in the fridge. The next morning, add chopped apple and chia seed.

If you would like to warm this up on the stove, add the chia seed after you heat it up. Do not boil!

Raw Sourdough Bread ★★★★

Ingredients:

2 ½ cups dry rye grain	2 ½ tsp caraway seeds
1 cup sunflower seeds	½ tsp Celtic sea salt (Redmond RealSalt™)
2 ½ tsp dill seeds	

Preparations:

Place 2 ½ cups of unsoaked rye grain (this yields 4 cups sprouted rye) in a large bowl with 4 cups of purified water and soak for 12-24 hours. Place 1 cup of sunflower seeds (this yields about 2 cups of sprouted sunflower seeds) into 3 cups of purified water and soak for 12-24 hours. Discard the water from the rye grains and the seeds. Evenly mix together all the ingredients in a large bowl.

Next, feed the ingredients through a juicer or blend in a Vitamix®. You will now have pliable bread dough. With your hands, knead the dough for a couple of minutes to blend all the ingredients evenly. Form the dough into a round ball and then flatten it to about 1 ½ inches thick, keeping the edges even.

Place the loaf on a mesh tray in a convection oven or dehydrator and dehydrate at 95°F for about 20-24 hours. The outside will be crusty and the inside moist. Store in a covered container in the refrigerator. Serves 5.

Poppy Seed Muffins ★★

Ingredients:

1   cup oat or spelt flour
2   tsp baking powder
¼   tsp salt
4   TBSP xylitol (Emerald Forest™)
½   cup cold water

1   tsp vanilla extract
¼   cup poppy seeds2   TBSP walnut oil
2   tsp orange oil
1   TBSP coconut oil

Preparations:

Preheat oven to 400°F. Oil 6-8 cups in a muffin tin with coconut oil. Sift together flour, baking powder, and salt. Stir in xylitol. Add water, vanilla, and poppy seeds. Mix until smooth, then stir in the walnut and orange oils. Pour into muffin cups. Bake for 25 minutes. Makes 6 to 8 muffins.

Carob Muffins ★

Ingredients:

⅓   cup pecans
1   cup boiling water
¼   cup walnut oil
¼   cup honey
2   eggs
1   tsp vanilla extract

1   cup spelt flour
⅓   cup carob powder
½   cup pecans, coarsely chopped
2   tsp baking powder
¾   tsp ground cinnamon
¼   tsp baking soda

Preparations:

Preheat oven to 350°F. Grind the ⅓ cup of pecans to a fine powder in a blender. Add boiling water and blend for 30 seconds, then add the walnut oil and honey and blend again. When cool, blend in the eggs and vanilla. Combine flour, carob, ½ cup chopped pecans, baking powder, cinnamon and baking soda in a large bowl. Mix well. Pour the liquid mixture into the dry ingredients and stir until well blended.

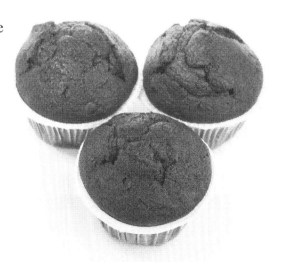

Bake in muffin cups for 25 minutes. Yields 8 muffins.

Fruit Bran Muffins *

Dry Ingredients:

1   cup oat bran
1   cup spelt flour
½   tsp sea salt (Redmond RealSalt™)
2   TBSP xylitol (Emerald Forest™)
1½ tsp baking powder
½   tsp baking soda
1   tsp cinnamon
1   tsp lemon zest
1   tsp xanthan gum (thickener)

Wet Ingredients:

1   can (8.5 oz.) crushed pineapple,
     drained, juice reserved
½   cup pineapple juice (from drained pineapple)
1   TBSP orange zest
½   cup orange sections, chopped
½   cup plain coconut or goat yogurt
½   cup coconut oil
2   egg whites, slightly beaten
1   tsp lemon juice
1   tsp vanilla extract

Preparations:

Preheat oven to 400°F. Use coconut oil to thoroughly grease 12 muffin cups. Blend together all the dry ingredients in a large bowl. Gently mix the wet ingredients together, except for the crushed pineapple. Add the dry ingredients to the wet. Stir the crushed pineapple into the batter with a few strokes; do not over mix. Spoon the batter into the prepared muffin cups, filling each ¾ full. Bake for 20 minutes. Serve warm. Yields 10-12 muffins.

Breakfast of Champions ★★★★

Ingredients:

1-2 cups cooked brown rice, sweet
     brown rice or spelt
juice of 1 lemon or lime
1   TBSP agave nectar (optional)
1-2 tsp flax oil
1-2 tsp liquid aminos (Bragg™)

½-1 avocado, chunked
2   TBSP sunflower seeds
2   TBSP almond slivers
1   firm tomato, chunked
1   tsp Spice Hunter's® Garlic
     Herb bread seasoning

Preparations:

Warm the rice up if you have time! Mix all ingredients except the bread seasoning together. Sprinkle the seasoning over the top. Serves 1-2.

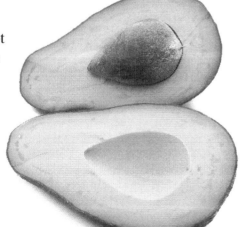

Cashew Butter Rolls ✶✶

Ingredients:

20 pitted dates
½ cup raisins
½ cup cashew butter

¼ cup chopped cashews
¼ cup sesame seeds coconut flakes,
    unsweetened

Preparations:

Blend the dates, raisins, and cashew butter together in a food processor or Champion Juicer™ with the screen plugged. Stir in the chopped cashews.

Form small amounts (about 1 TBSP) into rolls. Coat with sesame seeds and coconut flakes and store in the fridge or freezer for longer keeping. Makes 10-12 medium rolls.

My Mom's Puffed Pie ✶✶✶

Ingredients:

5 eggs
1 ¼ cup almond or coconut milk
1 tsp vanilla extract
1 ¼ cup spelt flour

¼ tsp sea salt (Redmond's RealSalt™)
1 tsp ground cinnamon
¼ tsp ground nutmeg
4 TBSP coconut oil

Preparations:

Preheat oven to 425°F. Beat the eggs. Add the milk and vanilla and stir until well combined. In a separate bowl, mix the flour, spices, and sea salt (Redmond's RealSalt™). Slowly stir the egg mixture into the dry mix until there are no lumps. Place the butter or coconut oil in a 4-quart casserole dish and then heat in the oven until it melts. Spread it evenly around the pan.

Pour the pancake mixture directly in the center of the dish and bake for 12-15 minutes. It will come out puffy. Serve with maple syrup, applesauce, or jam. Serves 4.

Fruit Verdé ✶✶✶

Ingredients:

25 fresh green grapes, halved
2-3 kiwi, chunked
1 pear, chunked

2 TBSP pineapple concentrate
2 TBSP coconut flakes

Preparations:

Cut up grapes, kiwi and pear and place together in a bowl. Gently stir in pineapple concentrate and coconut flakes. Serves 2.

Multi-Grain Cereal ★★★★

Tip: This is a great conventional cereal replacement. Reduce packaging waste and save bundles of money by buying bulk grains and using them in replacement. No need to have fortified vitamins as you get the real vitamins already in this recipe.

Ingredients:

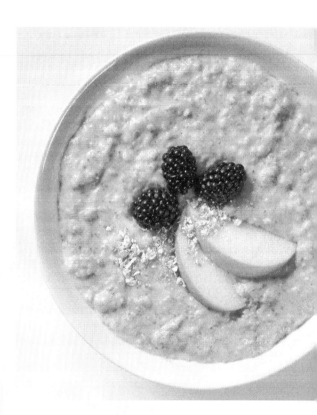

3 ½ cups water
½   cup oat groats
½   cup sweet brown rice
½   cup spelt
⅛   tsp cinnamon
pinch nutmeg
¼   tsp sea salt

Add after cooking:

¼   cup almond flakes
10 drops stevia (Sweet Leaf™)
1   cup coconut milk

Preparations:

Bring water to a boil, then add oat groats, brown rice and spelt. Turn to low and let simmer for 45 minutes. Strain out the water and add cinnamon, nutmeg, sea salt, almond flakes, and stevia.

Serve hot or cold with rice or almond milk.
Yields 3 ½ cups.

Fruit Smoothie ★★★★

Ingredients:

2 cups cold coconut milk (So Delicious™)
1 banana
1 cup berries (frozen)

½ avocado
1 cup spinach
2 dashes stevia (KAL™ or Sweet Leaf™)

Preparations:

Blend all ingredients until smooth. Serves 1.

Berry Blue Smoothie ★★★★

Ingredients:

1 cup blueberries
1 cup blackberries or raspberries
¾ cup coconut kefir (So Delicious™)
1 TBSP xylitol

1 dropper liquid stevia (optional)
½ cup water
½ banana
1 cup ice

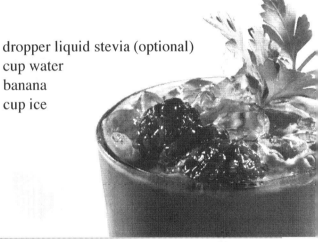

Preparations:

Blend all ingredients until creamy. Serves 1.

Walnut Raisin Breakfast Cake ★★

Tip: Arrowroot is a naturally healthy thickener and is available at any health food store.

Ingredients:

1 ⅔ cups water
½ cup raisins
½ pound pitted dates, chopped
⅓ cup coconut oil
2 tsp lemon juice

1 cup spelt flour
1 cup arrowroot powder
1 tsp baking soda
1 tsp ground cinnamon
½ cup walnuts, chopped

Preparations:

Preheat oven to 400°F. Combine water, raisins, and dates in a 3-quart saucepan. Boil for 10 minutes and set aside to cool. Stir together the oil and lemon juice in a medium bowl. Stir in the flour, arrow-root, baking soda, and cinnamon. Combine the flour mixture with the dates, raisins, and water in the saucepan. Mix well. Stir in the walnuts. Spread the batter into an oiled 8" or 9" square baking pan. Bake for 2 minutes, or until the top is firm when touched. Serves 8.

Brain Food ★★★

Ingredients:

½	cup coconut kefir (So Delicious™)	2	dashes ground nutmeg (optional)
1	TBSP cod liver oil (plain flavor)	2	dashes ground ginger
2	TBSP agave nectar	½	tsp rosemary powder
2	dashes ground cinnamon	½	tsp sage powder

Preparations:

Mix all ingredients together and drink. Serves 1.

Home Made Granola ★★

Note: When you soak nuts and seeds overnight it activates the sprouting process and increases the enzymes and amino acid content, thus making it twice as nutrient-dense.

Dry Ingredients:

4-5	cups rolled oats	¾	cup raw sunflower seeds
¾	cup wheat germ	½	cup almonds, slivered
½	cup bran or bran flakes (optional)	½	cup walnuts, chopped
½	cup sesame seeds	¾	cup flax seeds
¾	cup fresh or dried coconut		

Wet Ingredients:

¾	cup honey
2	tsp vanilla extract
⅓	cup apple juice

Preparations for Cooking Granola:

1. Mix all dry ingredients except the dried fruit in a large bowl. Mix wet ingredients separately, then pour over dry ingredients a little at a time, stirring to distribute evenly. Line a 9 x 13 inch baking pan with a thin layer of oil and arrange the mixture evenly in the pan.

2. Preheat oven to 300°F. For Cooking: Bake for one hour, stirring every 15 minutes. After removing from the oven, add dried fruit, cool to room temperature and store in airtight container.

Preparations for Raw Granola:

Follow the same steps in number 1 on previous page. Then place into the dehydrator with only the light on and allow to dehydrate for 10-12 hours or until dried. You can do this overnight so you can have the granola in the morning. Add the dried fruit after dehydrating. Serve with coconut milk or coconut kefir. Yields 10-11 cups.

A Berry Delicious Tart ★★★★

Tip: Agar-agar is tasteless seaweed used as a gelatin replacement.

Ingredients:

½	cup apple juice	2	ripe bananas
1½	TBSP agar-agar	2	ripe nectarines, sectioned and chunked
2	cups fresh strawberries, sliced	½	cup shredded coconut
2	cups fresh blueberries	¾	cup applesauce

Preparations:

Mix ½ cup apple juice with the agar-agar in a small saucepan and heat gently until dissolved, stirring constantly. Set aside to cool. Combine the fruits in a bowl. Blend the bananas and apple-sauce until smooth. Mix the banana/applesauce mixture with the apple juice/agar-agar and stir in the coconut.

Pour over the fruit. Mix gently. Pour into a bowl or decorative ring and chill until it sets. Serves 4.

Mediterranean Fruit Salad ★★★★

Ingredients:

¼	cup apple juice	4	dates, chopped
¼	cup raisins	½	avocado, chunked
1	banana, sliced		

Preparations:

Soak the raisins in the apple juice for 30 minutes. Combine all ingredients. Serves 2.

Oatmeal Pancakes ★★★★

Tip: Xylitol is a healthy sugar substitute, with half the calories of sugar, all of the taste, and it is safe for diabetics.

Ingredients:

¾   cup ground oats or oat flour
¼   tsp baking soda
1 ½ cups purified water
½   cup ground oats
1   TBSP xylitol (Emerald Forest™)

1   tsp baking powder
½   tsp sea salt (Redmond's RealSalt™)
3   TBSP coconut oil
2   TBSP purified water
1   tsp baking powder

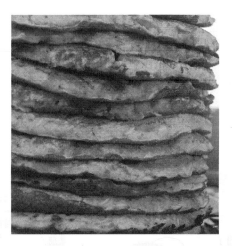

Preparations:

1. Combine ¾ cup ground oats, baking soda, and 1 ½ cups water; let stand for 5 minutes. Mixture will rise.

2. Separately combine ½ cup ground oats, xylitol, baking powder and salt.

3. Separately combine oil, water, and baking powder.
Mix ingredients in Steps 2 and 3 together first. Then add the ingredients in Step 1 and mix. Drop ¼ cup of this batter for each pancake onto a hot greased griddle.

Bake to a golden brown on each side. Yields 8-10 pancakes.

"BananOat" Waffles ★

Cheap Option: You can use water in place of coconut milk in this recipe. Make a bunch up at one time and freeze them. They taste great when toasted.

Ingredients:

2   bananas
4   cups rolled oats
1   pinch sea salt
½   cup coconut milk (So Delicious™)

½   cup water
1-2 TBS maple syrup or agave nectar
1   tsp vanilla
½   tsp sea salt (Redmond's RealSalt™)

Preparations:

Preheat a non-stick waffle iron to medium high. Place all ingredients in a blender in the order listed. Blend until thoroughly mixed. Pour batter in waffle iron and cook until golden brown (5-10 minutes).

Waffle Topping ★★

Ingredients:

2 peaches, finely chopped	3 TBSP juice or agave nectar
10 dates, finely chopped	2 pinches cinnamon
½ cup chopped nuts (walnuts or pecans)	

Preparations:

In a medium bowl, mix all items together and place on top of the waffles.

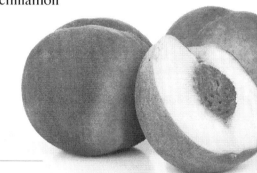

All American Fruit Salad ★★★★

Ingredients:

8 dates, chopped	3 ripe bananas, sliced
2 apples, chopped	2 ripe pears, chunked
¾ cup raisins	½ cup apple juice

Preparations:

Pour apple juice over the mixed fruit, cover, and refrigerate. Serve cold. Coconut flakes may be added if desired. Serves 2.

Charosset ★★

Tip: Charosset is a traditional Passover dish. It also makes for a great breakfast by itself or with toasted sprouted grain bread.

Ingredients:

3 apples, cored and grated	1 tsp ground nutmeg
1 cup walnut pieces	3 tsp lemon juice
¾ cup apricots, chopped	½ cup honey
1 TBSP lemon zest	½ cup raisins
1½ tsp ground cinnamon	4 TBSP sweet red wine or pineapple juice

Preparations:

Place all ingredients into a large bowl and mix well. Cover and chill. Serves 5.

All the Colors ★★

Ingredients:

2 oranges, segmented and chunked
½ pineapple, chunked
2 tangerines, segmented and chunked

1 grapefruit, segmented and chunked
1 pint strawberries, sliced
½ cup blueberries

Preparations:

Mix all fruits together. If additional juice is desired, add fresh squeezed orange juice. Serves 3.

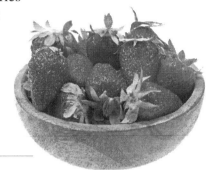

Raisin Victor Salad ★★★★

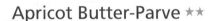

Ingredients:

1 apple, chunked
1 peach, chunked
2 bananas, sliced

¼ cup of raisins
3 cups red grapes, halved

Preparations:

Mix all fruits together and serve. Serves 3.

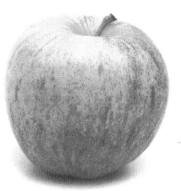

Apricot Butter-Parve ★★

Tip: any dried fruit can be used in this recipe.

Ingredients:

1½ cups dried apricots
½ cup almonds, whole

Preparations:

Soak the almonds and apricots in water overnight in separate containers. The next day discard the water and place the ingredients in a food processor using the "S" blade. Process the apricots and almonds to a smooth butter. Yields: 1½ cups. Keeps for up to 1 week in the refrigerator.

Vegan Quiche ✳✳✳

Ingredients:

¼	cup olive oil	4	cloves garlic, minced
1	onion, chopped	1	tsp dried basil
4	green onions, chopped	½	tsp pepper, divided 12 oz. firm tofu
	(separate the greens from the bottom)	⅛	cup liquid aminos (Bragg™)
2	medium potatoes, thinly sliced or cubed	4	TBSP nutritional yeast

Preparation:

Preheat oven to 325°F. In a large frying pan, sauté the onions, garlic, and bottoms of the green onions in olive oil for 2-3 minutes. Add potatoes, sea salt, and pepper, and sauté for 10-15 minutes, stirring occasionally until potatoes are golden brown. Blend tofu, liquid aminos, and nutritional yeast in a food processor or blender until well mixed. Mixture will be somewhat thick.
Add green onions and potatoes and pour into a greased pie pan. Cook 45-50 minutes, until top is firm and cooked all the way through. Sprinkle the top with goat cheese if desired, and enjoy!

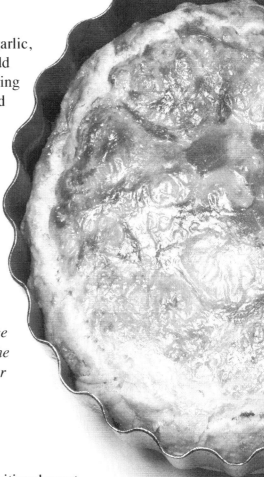

Vegetarian Quiche ✳✳✳✳

Options: If you don't have time to get a crust, no worries, you can make this recipe without one. In a pinch, I have used 1 piece of sprouted grain bread cubed and sprinkled on top of the quiche before baking. Also, ume plum vinegar can be used regularly for cooking, dairy free, as it adds a great salty cheese-like quality to dishes.

Ingredients:

1	cup coconut milk	1	tsp nutritional yeast
4	eggs	2	green onions, chopped
2-3	cups chopped or grated vegetables	½	tsp dill
2	cloves garlic, minced	2	tsp ume plum vinegar
¼	tsp sea salt	1	gluten-free pie crust (optional)
¼	tsp white or black pepper		

Preparations:

Preheat oven to 375°F. With a whisk or fork, mix together the coconut milk, eggs, vinegar, garlic, yeast, dill, salt, and pepper. The powdery substances will be a little lumpy but just mix as well as you can. They will dissolve while baking. Sauté the vegetables over medium heat for a few minutes until softened. If you are not using a crust, lightly oil the pie dish with coconut oil or another oil of your choice. Evenly place the vegetables in the dish, and then pour the liquids over the top until vegetables are covered evenly. Place into the oven and bake for 33-40 minutes. The quiche is done when you insert a knife in the center and it comes out clean. Since elevation can affect cooking time, add more time for elevations of more than 3,000 feet or check the doneness by inserting knife.

Soups, Salads, and Hors D'oeuvres

"Penicillin Soup" For Colds and Flu ★★★

The Food Beautiful lifestyle is centered around eating all plant-based nutrients. Like our ancestors, Food Beautiful believes that the occasional use of organic animal meat can be medicinal (like medicine). The occasional consumption of organic meats can alleviate sickness while preserving long-term health. If you get the flu or a cold it is best to drink soup broth so your energy is spent attacking the virus instead of digesting food. This speeds up your recovery time. If you are vegan or do not want to use chicken, make this with a vegetable-based broth, which in my opinion is just as effective, though different than what our ancestors used.

Ingredients:

1	4-5 lb. whole organic chicken with bones or just the bones	3	TBSP olive oil
1½	quarts boiling water	2	tsp sea salt
1	lb. onions, sliced into cubes	1	tsp fresh oregano, minced
1	large yam, peeled, cut in half crosswise	4-8	cloves garlic, minced
¾	lb. carrots, peeled, thickly sliced	4	TBSP parsley, minced
½	lb. parsnips, peeled, thickly sliced	1	tsp grated lemon peel
4	large celery stalks, cut into 2-inch pieces	3	TBSP lemon juice
		5	drops Stevia or 4 TBSP agave nectar (optional)

Preparations:

Quarter the whole chicken then cut each piece in two. Rinse the chicken well, leaving the skin on. Place the water into a large soup pot and bring to a boil. Add the chicken to the boiling water and allow boiling for 15 minutes then reduce the temperature to medium low. Prepare the onions, yams, carrots, parsnips, and celery stalks and set aside, keeping the onions separate from the other vegetables. Place the olive oil into a separate frying pan on medium high; allow the oil to come to a sizzle before adding all the onions and allow to simmer for 3 minutes. Remove the onions from frying pan and add to the chicken soup. After 1 hour of cooking the chicken add the vegetables, onions and sea salt to the chicken broth. Allow to cook on low for another 2 hours for a total time of 3 hours. About 10-15 minutes before the soup is done cooking, add the parsley, oregano and garlic. After the chicken broth is finished cooking, add the raw honey, lemon zest, and lemon juice. Allow to cool and discard the bones and skin.

Total cook time: 3 ½ hours. If you have children eating the soup remove the bones before serving. Makes 5-6 servings.

Digest Soup Ginger-Orange Butternut Squash Soup ✴✴✴

Ingredients:

2   TBSP coconut oil or olive oil
1   onion, finely chopped
⅓   cup chopped celery
2   TBSP grated fresh ginger or 1½ tsp ground ginger
3   lbs. butternut squash, peeled and cut into 1-inch chunks
1   small yam (such as Yukon Gold or Red Bliss), peeled and chopped

2   TBSP agave nectar or xylitol or 10 drops liquid stevia (optional)
4-5 cups vegetable stock
3   bags chamomile tea
½   cup orange juice (pulp removed)
2   tsp orange zest (grated orange peel)
sea salt and freshly ground white pepper
½   cup chopped chives and toasted nuts almond slivers (optional)

Preparations:

Bring 8 oz. water to a boil, add chamomile tea and let steep for 5 minutes. Remove the tea bags and squeeze out any excess liquid into the tea. In a large soup pot or Dutch oven, heat the coconut oil on medium; add onion, celery and ginger. Cook 5 minutes or until softened, stirring occasionally. Stir in the squash, yam, agave, vegetable stock, chamomile tea, orange juice, and zest. Season generously with salt and white pepper. Bring to a boil over high heat, then lower to a simmer. Cover the pot and cook for 40-60 minutes, until the squash is soft when pierced with a fork. Puree the soup in batches in a blender or with an immersion hand blender until very smooth. Garnish soup with chives and chopped toasted almond slivers. Serve warm. Serves 6-8.

"No More Constipation" Raw Creamy Spinach Soup ★★★★

Ingredients:

3   cups packed organic baby spinach
2   TBSP liquid aminos (Bragg™)
      or 1 tsp sea salt
2   cups hot water
2   cloves garlic, minced

1   ripe avocado
Juice of 1 lemon
2   TBSP agave nectar
¼   cup fresh cilantro or basil
2   TBSP psyllium or flax seed

Preparations:

Place all the ingredients in a food processor or Vitamix®. Turn machine on and begin pureeing ingredients while slowly pouring a thin stream of hot purified water into the food shoot. Stop when you have reached your desired creamy consistency. Allow to blend until all the chunks are gone. If you would like the soup warmer, place into a medium pot on medium low until the soup gets warm. Do not overcook, or the food will begin to lose its medicinal value.

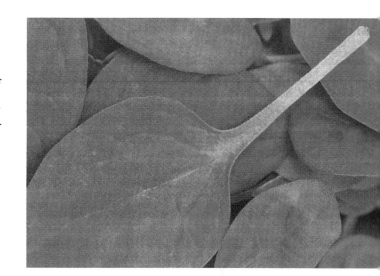

Strawberry Patch Soup ★

Tip: Goes well with Strawberry Pecan Salad.

Ingredients:

1   cup fresh strawberries, halved
½   cup xylitol (Emerald Forest™)
½   cup tofu sour cream (Tofutti™)
½   cup coconut milk (Nature's Forest™)

½   cup honey wine
4   mint leaves
¾   cup seltzer water

Preparations:

Combine strawberry halves, xylitol, sour cream, coconut milk, wine, half the pack of mint leaves, and seltzer water in a blender. Process until smooth. Pour into a medium large bowl and chill for 2-3 hours. To serve, ladle the soup into individual bowls and garnish with mint leaves, strawberries, and sour cream. Serves 4.

Tomato Soup for Eye Health ★★★★

Ingredients:

4	large, fresh tomatoes
1	cup unflavored coconut or hemp milk
2	tsp oregano
⅛	tsp stevia powder (Sweet Leaf™)

¾	tsp sea salt (Redmond's RealSalt™)
½	tsp thyme
2	tsp basil
1-2	TBSP olive oil

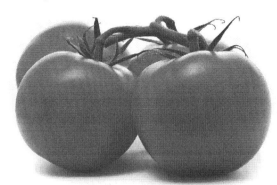

Preparations:

Pure all ingredients in blender, heat and serve.
Serves 2-3.

Caesar Salad ★★★★

Crouton Ingredients:

2	slices sprouted grain bread
1	TBSP extra virgin olive oil
2	tsp garlic sea salt (Redmond's RealSalt™)

Salad Ingredients:

1	head romaine lettuce
1	avocado, chunked
3	TBSP honey mustard
2	TBSP olive oil
2	TBSP liquid aminos (Bragg™)

Preparations:

Croutons: Cube the bread. Heat olive oil in a fry pan (on medium), spread evenly and add the bread cubes. Sprinkle with garlic salt. Toast on one side for 3 minutes. Add another TBSP of olive oil and flip. Sprinkle a little more garlic salt. Toast second side for 2 minutes. Remove from pan and cool.

Salad: Mash together the avocado, honey mustard, olive oil and liquid aminos in a large salad bowl. Cut romaine lettuce into bite-sized pieces and add to bowl with the dressing ingredients. Add croutons, toss and serve. Serves 2.

Kale Chips ★★★★

Ingredients:

1	bunch kale		sea salt to taste
4	TBSP coconut oil	1	tsp chili powder or garlic powder

Preparations:

Preheat the oven to 350°F. Cut the stems off the kale and discard; rinse and shake the leaves dry. Stack the leaves and cut them into 2 by 2 inch strips. Take the kale and place it into a deep bowl, then pour the coconut oil over top. Coat the kale on both sides.

Pull out a cookie sheet and thinly spread the kale over the cookie sheet so the leaves do not overlap. It is okay if they are slightly over lapped, just not on top of each other. Then evenly sprinkle on the sea salt, chili or garlic powder to desired taste. Roast the kale until some of the leaves looked tinged with brown, about 7 minutes. Take out and check to see if they are crispy enough. If they are brown do not cook them any further; if they are spongy cook them another 2 minutes. With a spatula lift the leaves off the cookie sheet and place them into a bowl for eating. Enjoy immediately.

Eggplant Rolls ★★★★

Tip: Use rice, almond, or vegan mozzarella cheese in this recipe if you have fungal-related issues or candida.

Ingredients:

1-2	large eggplant	2	tomatoes
3	TBSP olive oil	8	large fresh basil leaves
8	oz. rice, almond, vegan mozzarella, or raw goat cheese	4-6	TBSP prepared balsamic olive oil vinaigrette

Preparations:

Preheat oven to 400°F. Cut the eggplant into 8 slices lengthwise, then sprinkle salt on both sides and let sit for 20 minutes to draw out the bitter flavor. Rinse and pat dry. Place eggplant pieces on a large, oiled baking sheet. Drizzle the eggplant with vinaigrette dressing. Bake in oven for 8-10 minutes. Meanwhile, slice the tomato into ½ inch rounds and cut in half. Cut the cheese into ¼ inch, lengthwise slices. Place the cheese slices, tomato and basil leaves on the baked eggplant. Fold the eggplant over the filling. Broil for 3-4 minutes or until cheese melts. Serve warm. Yields 8-16 rolls.

Creamy Lentil Soup ★★★★

Ingredients:

1   cup green or brown lentils
32 oz. vegetable broth
2   cups water
1   medium yellow onion, finely chopped
1   tsp dried oregano
1   cup sweet brown rice, cooked
2   bay leaves

2   TBSP olive oil
½   tsp ground white pepper
1   tsp curry powder
1   tsp sea salt (to taste)
4   TBSP honey or xylitol
2   lemons and their peels,
      puréed in food processor

Preparations:

Rinse lentils in strainer until water runs clear. Place in a soup pot with the vegetable broth and water. Bring to a boil, lower to a simmer. Add bay leaves, oregano, pepper and curry powder. Cover and continue simmering for 25 minutes.

While the lentils are cooking, sauté onion in 2 TBSP olive oil until soft (about 5-6 minutes). Add the sautéed onion, cooked rice, and honey to the simmered lentils and spices. Continue cooking covered for another 20 minutes for a total cook time of 45 minutes. Finally, add the white pepper and puréed lemons and stir until evenly combined. Remove bay leaves and serve. For a creamier texture, blend all the ingredients in a blender and serve warm. Enjoy with spelt or rye crackers. Serves 5.

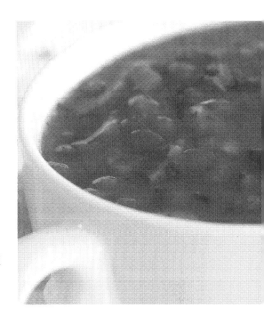

Simply Sweet Roasted Corn and Poblano Soup ★★★★

Ingredients:

12   ears sweet corn, cleaned
2   TBSP olive oil
salt and white pepper
½   gallon unsweetened coconut milk
½   gallon rich vegetable stock
4   TBSP coconut oil

2   red peppers, diced
1½   large white onions, diced
3   poblano peppers, diced
2   TBSP garlic, minced
3   jalapenos, minced

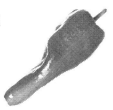

Preparations:

Preheat oven to 350°F. Cut corn from the cob, and place the cobs into a medium stock pot. Toss the corn kernels with the olive oil and season with the salt and white pepper. Spread evenly on a baking sheet and roast in the oven for 15-25 minutes until lightly browned. Add the coconut milk and vegetable stock to the cobs, bring to a boil then reduce to simmer for 30 minutes to 1 hour.

In a separate sauce pot, sauté red peppers, onions, poblano peppers, garlic, and jalapenos in the coconut oil until vegetables are just slightly cooked. Add roasted corn kernels and continue sautéing for another 2 minutes. Remove the cobs from the coconut milk and vegetable stock. Pour this broth over corn and vegetables. Simmer for 20 minutes. Strain out about a quarter of the vegetables and set aside. In a powerful blender, blend the soup a little at a time until very smooth. After the soup is puréed, add in the set aside vegetables for texture and color. Then season with sea salt and white pepper to taste. Serves 8.

Black Nile Salad ★★★★

Salad Ingredients:

½   cup quinoa
1   cup water
½   cube vegetable bouillon
1   cup sweet corn, organic
2   scallions, chopped
½   cup tomatoes, finely chopped
½   cup celery, thinly sliced
½   cup green peppers, chopped
1   can black beans, drained and rinsed

Dressing Ingredients:

3-4 TBSP olive oil
2   TBSP lemon juice
1   TBSP apple cider
2   cloves garlic, minced or pressed
1   tsp sea salt (Redmond's RealSalt™)
3   dashes stevia powder
1   tsp chili powder
1   tsp ground white pepper
2   TBSP each of fresh cilantro and parsley

Preparations:

Soak quinoa in water for five minutes, then drain or rinse thoroughly. Cook in water or vegetable bouillon and 2 TBS oil for 15-18 minutes on medium high heat. Allow to cool. Blend together all dressing ingredients.

Combine quinoa, corn, scallions, tomatoes, celery, peppers and black beans with dressing and mix well. For a spicier taste, add jalapeno peppers or a couple of dashes of cayenne. Serve cold. Serves 5.

RC-GC Salad ★★★

Tip: Look in Thai section of your health food store for sweet red chili oil.

Ingredients:

2 cups red cabbage, shredded
2 cups green cabbage, shredded
¾ cup raw cashews, chopped
4 TBSP honey or agave nectar
2 TBSP sweet red chili oil

1 TBSP lime or lemon juice
¼ cup cilantro leaves, finely chopped
1 tsp sea salt (Redmond's RealSalt™)
pepper to taste

Preparations:

In a saucepan, heat honey or agave nectar with the red chili oil. Add lime or lemon juice, cilantro, salt, and pepper. Combine with cabbage and mix well. Optional: lightly toast cashews in a dry fry pan on medium high heat for about 4-5 minutes and sprinkle on top of salad. Serve immediately or refrigerate and serve chilled. Serves 4.

Strawberry Pecan Salad ★★★

Citrus Dressing:

⅔ cup oil
¼ cup lime juice
2 TBSP orange juice
2 TBSP xylitol (Emerald Forest™)
⅛ tsp stevia (KAL™ or Sweet Leaf™) powder
1 tsp sea salt (Redmond's RealSalt™)
1 tsp lime zest
1 tsp orange zest

Salad:

8 cups romaine lettuce, chopped
1 red onion, thinly sliced
1 orange, chunked
1 pint strawberries, halved
2 avocados, thinly sliced

Topping:

¼ cup maple syrup (Shady Maple™)
⅔ cup pecans

Preparations:

1. Prepare pecans: Mix the pecans and maple in a small skillet and cook over medium heat until syrup gets thick and sticky (about 10 minutes).

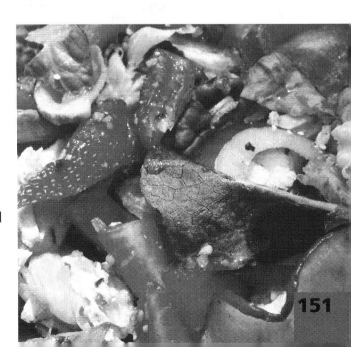

Cool for 10 minutes. The syrup should stick to the pecans. If it is still liquid after cooling, cook for another 5 minutes and cool again.

2. Prepare dressing: Combine the oil, lime and orange juice, xylitol, lime and orange zest, sea salt and stevia and shake in a jar. Chill until served.

3. Prepare salad: Toss the romaine, onion, orange chunks and strawberries in a large bowl and chill. When ready to serve, add the avocado slices and pecans and drizzle the dressing over the top. Serves 4-6.

Greek Salad ★★★★

Ingredients:

1	carrot, finely diced or grated	½	cup coriander leaves, chopped
2	cucumbers, finely diced	3	mint leaves, minced
2	onions, finely chopped	2	tsp fresh ginger, chopped
3	green chilies, finely chopped	4	TBSP agave nectar
1	tomato, finely diced		juice of 1 lemon
4	lettuce leaves, finely cut	1	tsp sea salt (Redmond's RealSalt™) or to taste
½	cup cabbage, shredded	1	cup prepared Greek dressing

Preparations:

Toss the carrot, cucumbers, onions, green chilies, tomato, lettuce, cabbage, coriander, mint and ginger together with sea salt. Combine the agave nectar and lemon juice and toss with vegetables. Add the Greek dressing and toss. Serve immediately or chill first. Serves 3.

Marinated Cucumber Salad ★★★★

Tip: ½ tsp of Stevia powder is equivalent to ½ cup honey or xylitol.

Ingredients:

2   medium cucumbers, thinly sliced
1   TBSP sea salt (Redmond's RealSalt™)
½   cup honey or xylitol
½   cup brown rice vinegar
1   TBSP apple juice
3   TBSP fresh dill, chopped
4   dashes white pepper

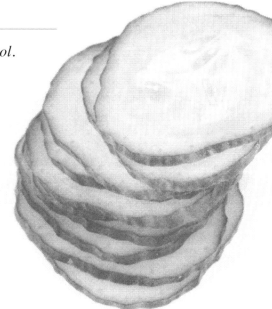

Preparations:

Layer thinly sliced cucumbers (with or without the skin) in a colander, sprinkling salt between each layer. Set the colander over a bowl large enough to catch the cucumber juice and let drain for 1 hour. Thoroughly rinse the cucumber slices under cold running water to remove excess salt. Pat dry with a cloth towel and set aside.

Gently heat the honey with the vinegar and apple juice until the mixture is thinned. Cool. Place the cucumbers into a bowl, pour the vinegar mixture over them and marinate for 2 hours. Drain and sprinkle with dill and pepper. Chill until ready to serve. Serves 5.

Rainbow Salad ★★★★

Ingredients:

1 cup red cabbage, grated	1 cup sprouts of choice
½ raw beet, grated	1 apple, grated
2 carrots, grated	1 cup pumpkin seeds
1 zucchini, grated	1 cup **Tahini Mint Dressing** (see recipe in Sauces section)
1 cup jicama, grated	
1 cup fresh green peas	

Preparations:

Toss all ingredients in a large salad bowl with Tahini Mint Dressing and serve. Serves 5.

Kung Pow Noodles ★★★★

Ingredients:

2 cups snow peas or early peas, slightly cooked
4 cups rice noodles, cooked, drained and cut into 2-inch lengths

Dressing Ingredients:

1 green onion, chopped
1 TBSP umeboshi paste
2-3 tsp dijon mustard
juice of 2 lemons
1-2 TBSP xylitol
1 TBSP sesame oil

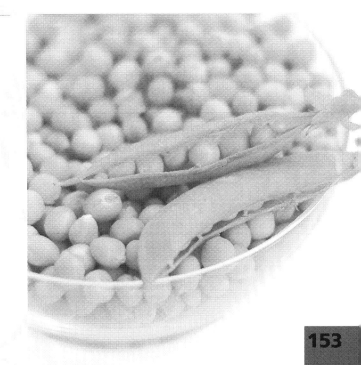

Preparations:

Combine the peas and noodles. Blend all dressing ingredients together and add to the noodle mixture. Mix lightly and serve before noodles become mushy. Serves 5.

Note: Umeboshi paste is made from a Japanese pickled plum and helps balance intestinal flora. This salad can help dissolve kidney stones, bladder and yeast infections.

Simple Sprouted Salad ★★★★

Ingredients:

2   cups alfalfa sprouts
2   cups mung sprouts
1   cup sunflower sprouts

1   cup lentil sprouts
1   cup **Avocado Lime Sauce** (see recipe in Sauces section)

Preparations:

On a plate, arrange an outside ring of alfalfa sprouts. Next make a ring of mung sprouts. Place sunflower sprouts in the center. Serve with your favorite salad dressing. Serves 2-3.

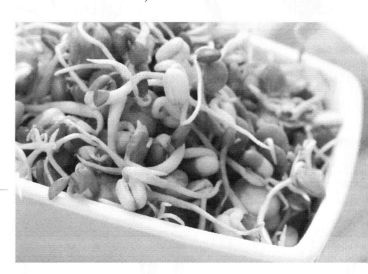

Rutabaga-Parsley Salad ★★★★

This salad can help dissolve kidney stones, bladder and yeast infections.

Ingredients:

1   cup salted, boiling water
½   bunch parsley
1-2 large rutabagas or turnips
1   tsp fresh ground horseradish
2   TBSP vegan mayonnaise (Follow Your Heart™)

¼   cup sauerkraut
pinch of stevia or 1 TBSP agave
½-1 tsp sea salt (Redmond's RealSalt™)

Preparations:

Plunge the parsley into salted boiling water for 3 minutes. Remove parsley, reserving the water. Finely chop the parsley. Cut rutabagas or turnips into round slices and cook in the parsley water (without the parsley) until tender. Mix the sauerkraut, stevia, salt, and mayonnaise together. Arrange the rutabagas or turnips over the bed of parsley and pour the dressing over the top. Serves 4.

Broccoli Pineapple Salad ★★

Ingredients:

2   bunches fresh broccoli, cut to bite-sized pieces
2   cups pineapple, cubed, or 2 cups apple, cubed
½   red onion, chopped
½   cup sunflower seeds
1   cup carrots, grated
1   cup vegan mayonnaise (Follow
     Your Heart™)

3   TBSP xylitol (Emerald Forest™)
2   TBSP apple cider vinegar (Bragg™)
2   dashes cayenne pepper
1   tsp sea salt

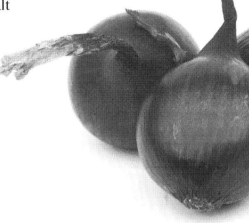

Preparations:

Mix all ingredients in a bowl and refrigerate for several hours.
Serves 5-7.

Low Carb Rolls ★★★★

*Note: If you want the cabbage leaves to be softer, dip them in hot water for a minute to soften.
Superb as a main-dish finger food when used with Reminiscent Peanut Sauce in the Salad Dressing
section!*

Ingredients:

8   green cabbage leaves
16   green leaf lettuce leaves, washed
     and dried
1   small bunch cilantro or basil, washed
     and dried

4   carrots, julienned
1   cucumber, julienned
8   leaves fresh mint
4   cups mung or bean sprouts
1   cup Reminiscent Peanut Sauce

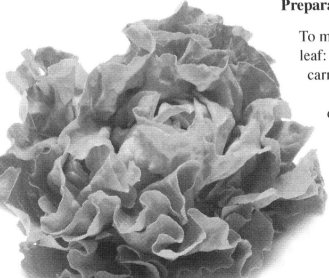

Preparations:

To make a roll, layer the following ingredients onto a cabbage
leaf: lettuce, Reminiscent Peanut sauce, cilantro,
carrots, cucumber, mint, and mung bean sprouts. Roll the
leaf, secure with two toothpicks, and cut in half on a
diagonal. Serve with extra Reminiscent Peanut Sauce.
Makes 8 rolls.

Kale Salad ★★★★

Note: Calamari figs are a brown color and slightly sweeter than Mission figs, which are purple. Both are readily found in health food stores. Figs help cleanse the colon wall of toxic debris. Any dark leafy green combines well with fruit.

Ingredients:

1	head kale, finely chopped	½	apple or mango, chopped
¼	cup fresh lemon juice	5	dried Calamari figs, finely chopped
⅛	tsp sea salt	1	dash stevia powder or 1 TBSP xylitol
½	avocado, diced	½	cup black olives, chopped

Preparations:

Finely chop the kale by rolling it up and slicing into 1/8 inch pieces. Place into a large bowl and massage the juice into the kale until it looks like it has been steamed. Add the other ingredients and mix thoroughly. Serves 4.

DELECTABLE SIDE DISHES

Mashed Potato Makeover ★★★★

Ingredients:

1 head cauliflower (steamed)
2 TBSP coconut oil or organic butter (to really imitate mashed potato flavor)
1 tsp sea salt

½ tsp black pepper (or to taste)
1 TBSP nutritional yeast (optional), adds a cheesy flavor

Preparations:

Steam the cauliflower until tender. Place into blender or food processor and add the coconut oil or butter, sea salt, black pepper and nutritional yeast. Blend until creamy.

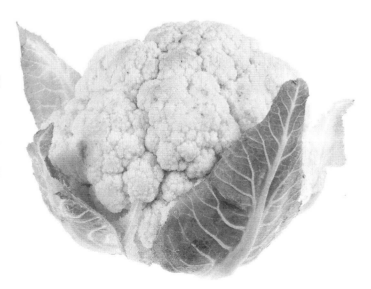

Sweet Potato Fries ★★★

Option: Cook in the oven for 15 minutes at 375, or until tender.

Ingredients:

2 large yams, peeled and cut in ¼ inch thick slices
3 TBSP coconut oil

1 TBSP ground rosemary
½ tsp sea salt (or to taste)

Preparation:

In a large skillet, on medium heat, heat the coconut oil over medium to high heat. Add yams and all remaining ingredients. Cover and cook over medium to low heat for 20 minutes or until yams are soft. Remove lid and toss the yams. Cook for another few minutes until all water is evaporated and yams are covered in sauce.

Red Curry Thai Dish ★★★★

Sauce Ingredients:

¾ cup lime juice
2 cloves garlic, minced or pressed
2 roasted red bell peppers, chopped
1 TBSP ginger root, chopped or pressed
2 TBSP fresh mint, chopped
¼ onion, chopped
1 tsp ground cumin

2-3 pinches ground cloves
cayenne pepper, to taste
¾ tsp paprika
14 oz. coconut milk (Nature's Forest™)
2 TBSP prepared red curry
½ cup honey

Other Ingredients:

4 cups brown rice, cooked
1 head broccoli, chopped into bite size pieces
1 zucchini, sliced in ¼ inch thick half rounds
2 carrots, sliced ¼ inch thick
½ head green cabbage, coarsely chopped

1 can Asian baby corn (Asian baby corn comes in tiny, whole cobs and is only available in jars or cans. Roasted red peppers come in jars as well.)

Preparations:

Cook the brown rice. Blend the lime juice, garlic, roasted bell peppers, ginger, mint, onion, cayenne, cumin, cloves, and paprika. Set aside. In a small saucepan, simmer the coconut milk, red curry sauce, blended herbs, and honey for 5 minutes. Steam the vegetables until lightly cooked but still crunchy. Top the rice with vegetables and sauce. Chicken also goes well with this dish! Serves 4.

Flax Crackers ★★★

Ingredients:

½ cup whole flaxseed	2 tsp cinnamon
2½ TBSP ground flax seed	3 TBSP agave nectar
4 TBSP coconut flakes (shredded)	½ cup warm water
1 TBSP chia seed	

Preparations:

Mix first five ingredients together in a medium size glass bowl. Add to this ½ cup warm and agave nectar, stir for 2-3 minutes until it thickens. Take a sheet of wax paper place on top of baking sheet. Spread a thin layer of flax seed--not too thin that you can see the wax paper through the flax seed. Using a pizza cutter, lightly score the flaxseed spread, into square shapes, so when it is finished you can snap it apart. Turn the light on in your oven (close the door) or turn on your dehydrator and place the flax spread inside. Dehydrate the crackers between 12-18 hours. To save yourself time and free up the oven for other uses, start dehydrating the crackers a couple hours before you go to bed. If they are still too soft allow them to dehydrate further. Makes 8 Large Crackers.

Basil Flax Crackers ★★★★

Ingredients:

5 cups carrot or vegetable pulp from juicing	¾ cup flax seed
2-3 cloves garlic crushed	1 TBS sea salt, or Braggs™ to taste
½ cup fresh basil, chopped -or- 3 TBS dried handful cilantro, chopped	2 ripe tomatoes, pureed
	¼ cup warm water

Preparations:

In a large mixing bowl combine the first five ingredients. Then add in the water and tomatoes mixing all the ingredients together so the ingredients are evenly distributed. Take a sheet of wax paper place on top of baking sheet. Spread a thin layer of flax seed--not to thin that you can see the wax paper through the flax seed. Using a pizza cutter, score lightly the mixture, into square shapes so when it is finished you can snap it apart. Turn the light on in your oven (close the door) or turn on your dehydrator and place the flax spread inside. Dehydrate the crackers between 12-18 hours. To save yourself time and free up the oven for other uses, start dehydrating the crackers a couple hours before you go to bed. If they are still too soft allow them to dehydrate further.

Green Curry with Halibut ★★★

Tip: You can make this sauce into a soup by adding more water during cooking.

Sauce Ingredients:

½ cup lemon juice
4   cloves garlic, minced or pressed
2-3 mild chiles, chopped
¼   onion, chopped
1   TBSP ginger root, pressed
2   dashes cayenne pepper
1   tsp ground cumin

2-3 pinches ground cloves
1   pinch cinnamon
14 oz. coconut milk
1-2 TBSP prepared green curry
½   cup honey
1   TBSP fish sauce (optional)
1   tsp sea salt

Other Ingredients:

2   halibut or cod steaks, 1 inch chunks
3-4 TBSP olive oil
1   head broccoli, chopped
1   zucchini, sliced in half rounds

2   carrots, sliced in rounds
½   head green cabbage, chunked
1   can baby corn, drained

Preparations:

Blend or process the lemon juice, garlic, chilies, onion, ginger, cayenne, cumin, cloves, and cinnamon. Set aside. In a large saucepan, simmer the coconut milk. Add the green curry sauce and honey. Stir in the blended herbs. Simmer and stir occasionally for 5 minutes. In a separate fry pan, heat 1 TBSP oil. Add fish, drizzle with 3 TBSP olive oil and sprinkle with 1 tsp sea salt (Redmond's Real-Salt™).

Continue cooking on stove, both sides, until fish flakes apart (about 8-10 minutes total). Steam vegetables until lightly cooked. Place the fish, drained corn, and steamed vegetables on a large, flat serving dish. Top with the sauce. Serves 3-4.

Sweet Potato Casserole ★★★★

Tip: Miso is a fermented brown rice or soy paste that is traditionally used in Japanese style meals and soups. It comes in three varieties with three intensities of flavor. White is sweet; red and brown is more. Azuki beans are known for their weight loss and cleansing properties. Black-eyed peas can be substituted for Aduki beans if desired.

Ingredients:

16 oz. can Azuki (or aduki) beans, drained
1   medium carrot, sliced
1   cup green beans, chunked
1   medium red onion, chopped
2   sweet potatoes or yams, cubed
½   cup peas
4   TBSP xylitol (Emerald Forest™)
4   TBSP olive oil or butter

½   cup rolled oats
2   tsp paprika
1   tsp dried thyme
1   TBSP white miso
3   TBSP tamari or liquid aminos (Bragg™)
¾   cup water
¾   cup coconut or almond milk

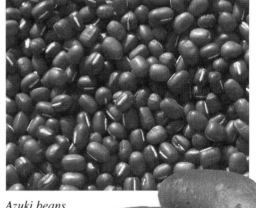

Azuki beans

Preparations:

Heat oven to 300°F. In a 2-3 quart casserole dish, dissolve miso with ¼ cup boiling water. Add aduki beans, stir in rolled oats, paprika, thyme, and liquid aminos. Add vegetables. Pour in water and coconut milk. Drizzle olive oil over all.

Bake, covered, for 1 hour and 35 minutes. Stir a couple of times during baking to make sure the mixture is not drying out. Add additional oil or almond milk if needed.

If it ends up too thin, add 1-2 TBSP ground flax seed, or ¼ tsp xanthan gum before serving. Serves 5.

Low Carb Casserole ★★★★

Ingredients:

4-5 collard green leaves, with course
    stem trimmed
3   cups broccoli, chopped
1   white onion, chopped
2   cloves garlic, minced or pressed
4   TBSP toasted sesame oil
4   TBSP xylitol (Emerald Forest™)
1   zucchini, sliced in half rounds
1   yam, cut in 1/8 inch thick slices

1   pkg. silken tofu
3   TBSP red palm oil
1   tsp thyme
⅛   tsp cayenne
1   tsp cumin
½   tsp sea salt (Redmond's RealSalt™)
2-3 TBSP honey
basil for garnish

Preparations:

Lightly steam the collard greens in ½ cup water until tender (about 3 minutes). Arrange evenly in a square baking dish. Slightly steam the yam slices for 3 minutes or until tender and set aside. Combine the broccoli, onion, garlic, sesame oil, and 2 TBSP of the xylitol in a food processor and process until chunky. (If you don't have a food processor, chop all the vegetables into the smallest size possible by hand.) Spread a layer of broccoli mixture over the steamed collard greens. Layer the zucchini slices over the broccoli mixture. Blend the silken tofu, red palm oil, 2 TBSP xylitol, cumin, cayenne, and sea salt together. Pour over the zucchini and greens. Place the slices of yam on top and drizzle with honey. Sprinkle with basil and serve. Serves 5.

Veggie Tortilla Wraps ★★★★

Ingredients:

4   cups firmly packed spinach
½   tsp liquid aminos (Bragg™)
½   tsp garlic powder
½   tsp paprika
2   dashes cayenne (optional)
2   dashes ground white pepper
½   tsp sage
2   TBSP olive oil

4   oz. pepper jack Rice cheese, grated
¾   cup black beans or pureed black beans
1   cup carrots, grated
1   cup sprouts of choice (lentils or alfalfa)
½   cup prepared chili sauce (optional)
2   TBSP goat yogurt (optional)
2   sprouted grain tortillas

Preparations:

Take the spinach and in a small bowl massage it down so it looks like it has been steamed. Add the next seven ingredients to the spinach. In order place a couple slices cheese, beans, spinach and sprouts in the middle of each tortilla. Top with carrots, goat yogurt and chili sauce.

Option: For a warm tortilla: Heat up the black beans in a small pan. Put the filled tortillas in a pan with 1 TBSP coconut oil, over medium heat for 2 minutes on each side. Top with the chili sauce to taste.

Tip: Put a plate overtop the tortilla while it is heating, which keeps it from opening up. Makes 2 tortillas.

African Pineapple Moussaka ⋆⋆

Ingredients:

1 cup onions, chopped	1 TBSP tabasco or hot pepper sauce
2 cloves garlic, minced or pressed	3 TBSP honey
1½ TBSP coconut or olive oil	½ cup cilantro, chopped
4 cups kale, sliced	2 tsp sea salt
2 cups pineapple (fresh is best), chunked	½ tsp mint
½ cup almond butter	

Preparations:

Wash the kale and remove stems. Roll leaves and cut into 1 inch wide slices and set aside. In a covered saucepan, sauté the onions and garlic in the oil for about 10 minutes, stirring frequently, until the onions are lightly browned.

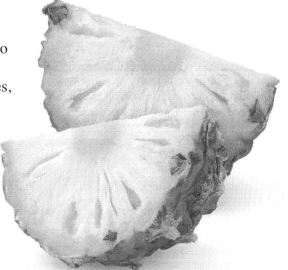

Add the pineapple to the onions and bring to a simmer. Stir in the kale, cover, and return to simmer for about 5 minutes, stirring a couple of times, until just tender. Mix in the almond butter, hot pepper sauce, sea salt, mint, cilantro, and honey. Simmer for 5 more minutes. Serve warm and enjoy with toasted, sprouted wheat bread. Serves 5.

Tempe and Cauliflower Explosion ★★★★

Tip: You can substitute a half pound of shredded, cooked chicken for the tempe. Drain the water from the tofu. Rinse with cold water. Slice into 1 inch slices; lay on a cookie sheet between clean towels, top with another cookie sheet and weight with a large book.

Ingredients:

2	TBSP toasted sesame oil	⅛	cup jalapeno peppers, sliced
½	lb. extra firm tempe, pressed and cubed	1	tsp cumin
2-3	tsp curry powder	1	tsp sea salt (Redmond's RealSalt™)
4	cloves garlic, minced or pressed	½	tsp cracked white pepper
½	head cauliflower, cut into florets	3	dashes stevia
½	onion, quartered and sliced	2	tomatoes, fresh diced, or 1 can
1	can chickpeas (garbanzo beans), drained		diced tomatoes

Preparations:

Heat toasted sesame oil over medium high heat. Add the crushed garlic. Add tofu cubes, sprinkle with curry and let brown on one side. Flip each piece of tofu, sprinkle again with curry and let cook for 1 minute. Add the cauliflower and onions and sauté for 5 minutes, stirring occasionally. Add the garbanzo beans, cumin, sea salt, stevia, and white pepper, mixing thoroughly. Cover and simmer for about 10 minutes. Add the tomatoes and simmer for another 5 minutes, covered. Serves 5.

Broccoli and Tempe in Garlic Sauce ★★★★

Ingredients:

2	cups brown rice, cooked	1½	tsp ground ginger
2	TBSP olive or sesame oil	¼	tsp cayenne pepper
2	lbs. broccoli florets	⅓	cup liquid aminos (Bragg™)
8	oz. tempe, cubed	3	TBSP corn starch or ¼ tsp xanthan gum
1	medium onion, diced	3	dashes stevia
3	TBSP garlic, crushed or minced	½-1	cup water

Preparations:

Sauté the onion and garlic in olive or sesame oil on medium heat until the onion begins to turn translucent. Add the broccoli, tofu, ginger, and cayenne pepper and stir fry until the broccoli is tender. Mix the corn starch (or xanthan gum), stevia, and liquid aminos with about ½ cup of the water. Add to the broccoli and tofu. Continue cooking and mixing until the sauce thickens and all the ingredients are thoroughly coated. Add additional water as necessary to thin the sauce. Serve over a bed of brown rice. Serves 5.

Vegan Spicy Chili ★★★★

Tip: This chili recipe can be made with one kind of bean or several varieties (black, kidney, pinto, or multi-bean blends). The chili can be prepared in a crock pot (slow cooker) or in a large covered pot on the stove.

Ingredients:

2 lbs. mixed dry beans (black, pinto, kidney)	2 TBSP minced garlic
2 lbs. fresh tomatoes	2 TBSP chili powder
1 large onion, diced	2 TBSP cumin
1 lb. extra firm tofu, cubed (optional)	1 TBSP dried basil
1 lb. corn	5 TBSP olive oil or butter
1 green bell pepper, diced	2-3 chipotle peppers, chopped
¼ tsp stevia or ½ cup xylitol (Emerald Forest™)	¼ tsp cayenne pepper (optional)

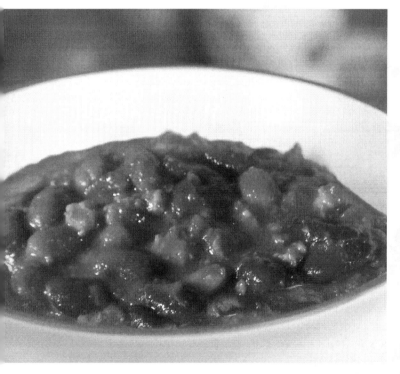

Crock Pot Preparations:

The night before, wash the beans and place in crock pot with 10 cups of boiling water. Cook on high until you're ready for bed; turn the crock pot to low for overnight. First thing in the morning, turn the crock pot to high, add all the other ingredients and cook for another 4 to 6 hours. Add water as necessary.

Stove Top Preparations:

The night before, wash the beans and place in a large, covered pot with 10 cups of water and soak overnight. First thing in the morning bring the water to a boil, and then simmer the beans for 35 minutes. Add all the other ingredients, return to a boil, then lower the heat to a simmer for another 4 to 6 hours. Stir often during the cooking process. If the chili begins to thicken before it is thoroughly cooked, add a little water. Serve the chili alone, over brown rice, or with a fresh salad. Use the leftovers to make a chili salad. Serves 5.

Simplest Veggie Burgers ★★★★

Note: Vegan Bean Burger option: omit the egg. Add ½ cup mashed potatoes.

Ingredients:

2   cups well-cooked black beans, drained
1   medium onion, quartered (sauté or leave raw)
½   cup rolled oats (preferably not instant)
1   TBSP chili powder
1   tsp sea salt

3   eggs or ½ cup mashed potatoes
½   tsp ground white or black pepper
3-5 TBSP bean-cooking liquid, if
      needs more liquid
coconut oil (for cooking)

Preparations:

1. Combine the beans, onion, oats, chili powder, salt, pepper, and egg in a food processor and pulse until chunky but not puréed, adding a little liquid if necessary to produce a moist but not wet mixture. Let the mixture rest for a few minutes if time allows.

2. With wet hands, shape into whatever size patties you want and again let rest for a few minutes if time allows. (You can make the burger mixture or even shape the burgers up to a day or so in advance. Just cover tightly and refrigerate, then bring everything back to room temperature before cooking.) Film the bottom of a large nonstick or well-seasoned cast-iron skillet with oil and turn the heat to medium. A minute later, add the patties. Cook until nicely browned on one side, about 5 minutes; turn carefully and cook on the other side until firm and browned.

3. Serve on buns with the usual burger fixings. Or cool and refrigerate or freeze for later use.

Dense Veggie Burgers ★★★★

Tip: Chick pea flour can be purchased in a health food store. This recipe will make 12 veggie burgers. Enjoy on spelt or sprouted grain buns with sliced tomatoes, romaine lettuce, mustard, and fruit-juice sweetened ketchup.

Ingredients:

1   cup brown rice, uncooked
1   cup lentils, dry
4½ cups water
1   cup chick pea/garbanzo flour
1   cup oat flour, or quick oats
1   TBSP sea salt
6   oz. tomato paste
3   medium carrots, shredded

1   medium potato, shredded
1   medium onion, finely chopped
4   cloves garlic, minced or pressed
1   TBSP oregano
2   chipotle peppers, finely chopped,
    or 1 tsp smoke flavor
hot pepper sauce, to taste
corn meal

Burger Preparations:

1. Cook the rice and lentils: Boil water in a medium sized, covered pot. Add the brown rice and lentils return to a boil then reduce the heat to a simmer and cook until all the water is absorbed, about 45 minutes.

2. Combine: Put the brown rice and lentils into a large mixing bowl, add the tomato paste and thoroughly mash together. Then add all the shredded/chopped vegetables and continue mashing together with a potato masher or your hands. Add ¼ cup of the chick pea flour and oat flour (or quick oats) and continue mashing. Continue to add the flour in ¼ cup increments until all the ingredients are completely blended.

3. Bake: Preheat oven to 350°F. Thoroughly dust the surface of a large baking sheet with corn meal. Form the mix into the desired "burger" size and place on the baking sheet. Bake for 75 minutes (for slightly crispy burgers) or 55-60 minutes (for softer burgers). Enjoy with sprouted grain buns, sliced tomatoes, romaine lettuce, and fruit juice-sweetened ketchup. Serves 5-7.

Taco Stackup ★★★★

Ingredients:

2 cups brown rice, cooked	1 avocado, cubed
4 cups shredded lettuce	½ cup rice cheese, mozzarella, grated
2 cup zucchini, grated or chopped	3 oz. organic corn chips
1½ cup black beans, cooked	½-¾ cup **Avocado Lime Sauce** (dressing section)

Preparations:

Pull out a plate and layer in order the first 5 ingredients, then pour over the avocado lime sauce and top with crushed chips. Serves 2.

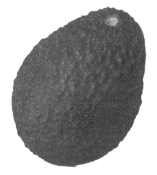

Power Pack Wrap ★★★★

Ingredients:

1 sprouted grain tortilla wrap	1½ cups tightly packed spinach
2-3 TBSP hummus	1-2 TBSP Vegenaise® (Follow Your Heart®)
1½ cups sprouted lentils	1 TBSP liquid aminos (Bragg™)
1 TBSP chopped sunflower seeds	2 cloves garlic, crushed

Preparation:

Lay out 1 sprouted tortilla wrap. Evenly spread hummus in the middle of tortilla. In a separate bowl, massage the spinach 30 seconds, until it looks like it is steamed. Then add the Vegenaise, liquid aminos, and garlic to the spinach and mix together.

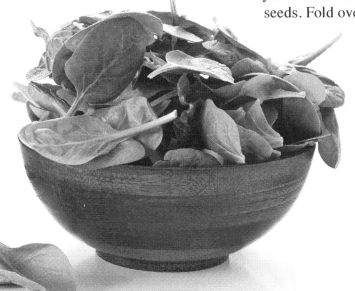

Layer in order inside: sprouted lentils, spinach cream, sunflower seeds. Fold over and use a tooth pick to keep wrap together. If you would like, you can warm up the tortilla on the stove top before adding the fillings. Eat fresh and enjoy. Serves 1.

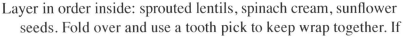

Lentil Loaf with Barbecue Sauce ★★★

Tip: Serve this cold as the perfect meat substitute on sandwiches with avocado, sliced tomatoes, and onions.

Ingredients:

1½ cups lentils, uncooked	½ cup hot sauce (to taste)
3½ cups water	2 TBSP unsulphured molasses
1 tsp sea salt (Redmond's RealSalt™)	1 TBSP brown mustard
1 cup brown rice, uncooked	1 TBSP liquid aminos (Bragg™)
2 cups water	2 cloves garlic, minced or pressed
2 onions, finely diced	2 tsp sage
4 TBSP olive oil	1 tsp marjoram
6 TBSP tomato puree	2 TBSP xylitol

Preparations:

1. Cook the lentils: Place 3 ½ cups of cold water in a covered pot and bring to a boil. While the water is heating, rinse the lentils in a strainer and remove any stones or other foreign matter. Add the rinsed lentils and sea salt to the boiling water turn to low and allow to simmer. Cook until all the water is absorbed.

2. Cook the rice: Place 2 cups of cold water in a covered pot and bring to a boil. Add the rice, cover, and lower the heat to a simmer. Cook until all the water is absorbed (about 50 minutes).

3. Sauté the onions: While the lentils and rice are cooking, finely dice the onions and sauté in 2 TBSP of the oil for 2-3 minutes. Add the onions to the lentil pot before the water is completely absorbed and continue cooking until the water is all absorbed.

4. Prepare the barbecue sauce: In a small mixing bowl, thoroughly combine 2 TBSP olive oil, tomato puree, hot sauce, molasses, mustard, liquid aminos, and one half of the garlic, sage, marjoram, and xylitol.

5. Prepare the mixture: When all the water has been absorbed in the pot of lentils and onions place them in a large mixing bowl and coarsely mash so that most of the lentils are broken. Add the other half of the garlic, sage, marjoram, onion, xylitol and one half of the barbecue sauce to the mashed lentils and mix well. Add the cooked rice and, again, mix thoroughly!

6. Bake the loaf: Preheat oven to 350°F. Firmly press the mixture into a lightly oiled loaf pan or ceramic baking dish. Pour on the remaining barbecue sauce and spread evenly over the surface. Bake for 1 hour.

7. Serve: Cut into ½ inch slices and serve open faced with toasted, sprouted wheat bread and slices of tomato and onion. Add fruit juice-sweetened ketchup or vegan mayonnaise for extra flavor. Serves 8.

Delish Lasagna ⋆⋆⋆

Tip: This vegetarian lasagna is dairy-free, meat-free, wheat-free, and sugar-free. All of the flavor, none of the guilt! Food Beautiful usually recommends eating spinach raw as cooked spinach can have high amounts of oxalic acid that can crystallize in the joints. Feel free to substitute the spinach in this recipe with kale.

Ingredients:

4	zucchini, sliced thin lengthwise	1	tsp ground white pepper
3	lbs. spinach or kale, coarsely chopped	1	tsp sea salt (Redmond's RealSalt™)
1	qt. spaghetti sauce	4	dashes stevia (KAL™ or Sweet Leaf™)
2	TBSP olive oil	¼	tsp cayenne pepper
1	large onion, diced	1	lb. brown rice lasagna noodles
2	TBSP garlic, minced or pressed	1	lb. firm tofu
2	tsp dried oregano	½	cup lemon juice
2	tsp dried sweet basil	⅔	cup nutritional yeast
1	tsp ground fennel	3	TBSP corn starch or 1 tsp xanthan gum

Preparations:

Preheat oven to 350°F

1. Prepare the sauce: In a medium size pot, sauté the diced onions in olive oil until transparent, then add the spaghetti sauce, spices, stevia, and sea salt and bring to a simmer for 3 minutes. Add the spinach or kale. Continue cooking until the sauce returns to a simmer. Remove from heat and set aside.

2. Prepare the noodles: While the spinach or kale is cooking, follow the directions on the box to cook the lasagna noodles until tender. Rinse with cold water and set aside.

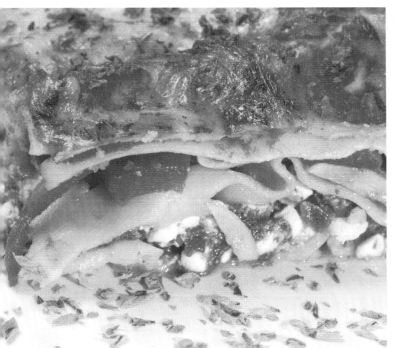

3. Prepare the tofu sauce: Place the tofu, lemon juice, nutritional yeast, and cornstarch into a blender or food processor and blend at high speed until creamy.

4. Prepare for baking: In a 2-quart glass baking dish, place a layer of the tomato/spinach sauce, a layer of lasagna noodles, a thin layer of the tofu sauce, and a layer of zucchini. Repeat layering in the same order until all the ingredients are used or until the baking dish is full. Try to have at least three sets of layers. Bake in the oven for 30-35 minutes. Cool for about 10 minutes before serving. Serves 6.

Asian Stir-Fry ⋆

Ingredients:

2 TBSP fruit-sweetened ketchup (Muir Glen Organics™)
1-2 TBSP xylitol (Emerald Forest™)
2 TBSP liquid aminos (Bragg™)
2 TBSP sunflower or olive oil

1 lb. carrots, julienned
2 leeks, julienned
2 oranges, segmented
1 cup cashews or almonds, chopped

Preparations:

Mix the fruit-sweetened ketchup, xylitol, and liquid aminos together in a small bowl and set aside. Heat the oil in a large wok or frying pan until it begins to sizzle. Add the carrots leeks and stir-fry (high heat) for 2-3 minutes or until vegetables are softened. Turn down the heat, add the orange segments and heat through gently for 2 minutes, being careful not to break them as you stir. Add the liquid aminos/ketchup mixture to the wok and cook for 2 more minutes. Transfer the stir-fry to warm serving bowls and sprinkle with cashews or almonds and serve immediately. Serves 5.

Zucchini Curry Pasta ⋆⋆⋆

Tip: This vegetable mixture also goes well over brown rice.

Ingredients:

1 large onion, coarsely chopped
1½ TBSP garlic, minced or pressed
3-4 medium carrots, sliced
1 cup raisins
2 TBSP olive oil
2 medium zucchini, sliced
1 medium yellow squash, sliced
28 oz. can crushed tomatoes
1 cup walnuts, large pieces
1 TBSP ground turmeric

1 TBSP paprika
2 tsp sea salt (Redmond's RealSalt™)
4 TBSP honey
1½ tsp ground cinnamon
¼ tsp cayenne pepper
1 TBSP cumin, ground
3 fuji apples, cut in ¼ inch chunks
1 lb. kamut penne pasta (Eden Organics™)
2 TBSP olive oil

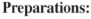

Preparations:

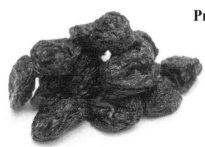

Heat 2 TBSP olive oil in a large fry pan or wok and cook the onion, garlic, carrots, and raisins on medium heat until the onions turn translucent. Add the zucchini and yellow squash, tomatoes, walnuts and all the spices until the vegetables are tender (about 10

minutes). Stir as necessary to ensure uniform cooking. Add the apples and cook slightly longer until tender, but not mushy.

Cook the kamut penne pasta according to package directions. Strain and add 2 TBSP of olive oil, so the noodles won't stick together. In a large serving bowl, combine the pasta and vegetable mixture. Serve warm or cold. Serves 5-7.

California Pizza with Spelt Crust ★★

Tip: Pre-made spelt pizza crusts are available at most health food stores.

Pizza Crust Ingredients:

1 TBSP active dry yeast	2 TBSP honey or ½ dropper liquid stevia (KAL™ or Sweet Leaf™)
1¼ cups warm water	
2 TBSP brown rice flour	1 tsp sea salt (Redmond's RealSalt™)
2 TBSP sunflower or olive oil	3½ cups spelt flour

Preparations:

Mix ¼ cup warm water and yeast in a small bowl and set aside. Mix 1 cup warm water, brown rice flour, oil, honey or stevia, and sea salt in a large mixing bowl. When yeast is soft and bubbly stir it into this mixture as well. Add 1½ cups of flour to the mixture and beat together well. Add more flour gradually until dough is no longer sticky and there are no lumps. Turn the dough onto a floured board and knead for 10 minutes, adding flour as needed to keep the dough from sticking to the board. Return the dough to a clean, oiled bowl and let rise in a warm place for 1 hour. While the dough is rising, prepare the other ingredients. Makes two 9" crusts, or one 18" crust.

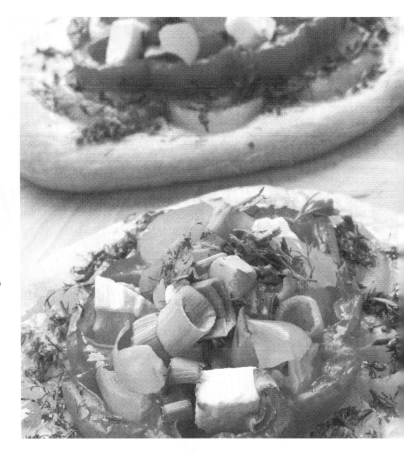

Pizza Toppings Ingredients:

1 cup tomato sauce	6 slices tomato (optional)
1-2 TBSP olive oil	1 tsp oregano
1 medium onion, chopped	1 tsp basil
8 oz. sliced olives	½ tsp thyme
1½ cup zucchini, grated	¼ tsp white pepper
½ cup pine nuts (optional)	2 cups shredded cheese substitute
3 cloves garlic, minced or pressed	(soy, rice, or almond) or raw cheese

Preparations:

When dough has risen, preheat oven to 400°F. Oil one large or two small cookie sheets or pizza pans generously with olive oil. Heat pans in the oven for a minute while you roll out the dough. Roll or stretch the dough to fit the pan(s). Cover with tomato sauce (if you can't use tomato sauce, spread crust with ¼ cup prepared red chili sauce or use another sauce of choice). Sprinkle sea salt and all other spices over sauce. Evenly spread vegetables, and then add shredded cheese. Garnish with tomatoes and drizzle with olive oil. Bake for 15 minutes or until crust is brown. Yields 2 pizzas.

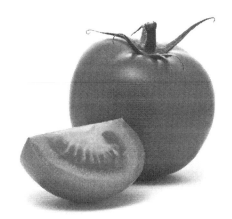

Mediterranean Pasta ★★★

Ingredients:

2 large eggplants	4 TBSP maple syrup
¼ cup olive oil	2 TBSP capers, drained (optional)
1 tsp sea salt (Redmond's RealSalt™)	1 can black olives, sliced
2 cloves garlic, minced or pressed	4 TBSP fresh parsley, finely chopped
1 tsp ground white pepper	½ tsp sea salt (Redmond's RealSalt™)
2 lemons, juiced	1 lb. brown rice rotini noodles
½ tsp lemon zest	

Preparations:

Cut eggplant into 1-inch cubes, place in a colander and sprinkle with sea salt. Let stand for 30 minutes to remove the bitter flavor. Rinse and pat dry with a cloth towel. Heat the olive oil, sea salt, garlic, and pepper in a large frying pan. Sauté the eggplant cubes over medium heat for 8-10 minutes, tossing regularly, until golden brown and softened (you may need to do this in two batches to ensure all of it gets cooked.) Place the eggplant in a large serving bowl and toss with the lemon juice, lemon zest, maple syrup, capers, olives, sea salt, parsley, and grated lemon rind.

Cook noodles according to package directions; drain and rinse. Mix together with all other ingredients. Serve warm or cold. Serves 4-5.

Roasted Baby Vegetables ★★★★

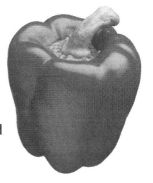

Vegetables:

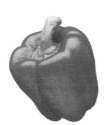

1 eggplant, sliced	2 cups mushrooms, sliced
1 red onion, sliced	1 cup grape tomatoes
2 zucchinis, sliced	2 red bell peppers, chunked

Dressing:

½ cup olive oil
1 tsp parsley
1 tsp rosemary
1 tsp thyme
½ tsp white pepper

4 dashes stevia powder
3 cloves garlic, minced or pressed
1½ tsp sea salt
4 TBSP BBQ sauce

Preparations:

Preheat oven to 400°F. In a small bowl, mix the olive oil, herbs, and BBQ sauce. Oil 2 large cookie sheets with sides. Spread the vegetables on the sheets in a single layer and top with the oil herb mixture. Bake for 10 minutes or until the vegetables are tender. Serves 4-5.

Asparagus Egg Tart ★★

Ingredients for piecrust:

6 TBSP butter or coconut oil
1½ cup spelt flour

pinch sea salt (Redmond's RealSalt™)
¼ cup cold water

Ingredients for filling:

8 oz. asparagus
3-4 eggs, beaten
1 cup pepper jack rice (or goat) cheese

3 TBSP plain goat yogurt
sea salt
white pepper to taste

Preparations:

Preheat oven to 400°F. In a bowl, combine the flour and salt. Cut the butter into the flour mixture. Stir in ¼ cup cold water to form smooth dough. Knead lightly on a floured surface for a few minutes. Roll out the dough to fit a 9-inch pie pan. Press rolled dough into the pan and pinch the edges. Bake for 10 minutes until it is firm but still pale.

Reduce oven temperature to 350°F. Trim each asparagus stalk 2 inches from the top and set these pieces aside. Cut the remaining asparagus into 1-inch pieces. Beat the eggs, mix in the yogurt or kefir and grated rice or goat cheese. Stir in the asparagus stalks and pour into the pastry shell. Place the asparagus tips on top. Bake for 35-40 minutes or until golden. Serve hot or cold. Yields 4-8 slices.

Maple Nut Squash *

Ingredients:

1 acorn squash	¼ tsp ground cloves
1 cup onions, finely chopped	½ tsp sea salt
½ cup walnuts, pieces	4 TBSP maple syrup
½ cup raisins	1 cup brown or basmati rice
1 tsp ground cinnamon	2 cups water
½ tsp ground ginger	

Preparations:

Preheat oven to 375°F. Wash the squash and cut in half lengthwise. Scoop out the seeds (can be saved for roasting) and bake in a covered roasting pan for 55 minutes. Meanwhile, boil 2 cups of water in a covered pot. Add the rice, spices and sea salt and simmer for 40 minutes. Add the onions, walnuts, and raisins and continue cooking for 10 more minutes.

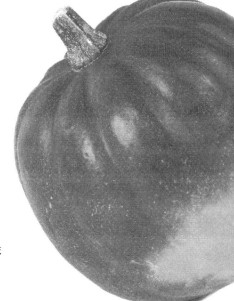

When the rice mixture is cooked and the squash has baked for 55 minutes, spoon the rice into each of the holes in the squash and continue baking for an additional 15 minutes. Allow to cool for 10 minute before serving. Serves 3.

Stuffed Butternut and Walnut Squash *

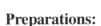

Ingredients:

1   butternut squash
1   apple, chunked
½   cup dried apricots, diced
½   cup pecans, chopped

4   TBSP maple syrup
2   tsp ground cinnamon
1   tsp sea salt

Preparations:

Preheat oven to 400°F. Wash the squash and cut in half lengthwise. Scoop out the seeds and pierce the skin on each side 4-6 times with a fork. Place the squash in a glass baking dish with 1 inch of water. Bake for 1 hour.

Meanwhile, combine the apple, papaya, pecans, maple syrup, and cinnamon, and mix well. After the squash has baked for 1 hour, fill each cavity with the apple mixture, cover and bake for another 30 minutes, or until the center of the squash is tender. Cool for 15 minutes and serve with roasted lamb or oven roasted turkey. Serves 3.

DESSERTS

Chocolate Crêpe With Strawberry Walnut Filling *

Crêpe Ingredients:

3   TBSP cocoa powder or
    carob powder or 2 oz. baker's chocolate
½   TBSP cardamom
2   TBSP maple syrup (Shady Maple™)
1½ cups almond milk

3   eggs, beaten
½   TBSP baking soda
1   cup brown rice flour
3   TBSP xylitol (Emerald Forest™)
3   TBSP butter or oil

Filling Ingredients:

4   cups fresh strawberries, sliced
5   TBSP maple syrup (Shady Maple™)
1   TBSP coconut oil

½   cup walnuts, chopped
3   TBSP coconut milk
½   tsp xanthan gum

Crêpe Preparations:

Melt butter, 2 TBSP cocoa powder, cardamom, and maple syrup in saucepan, stirring while butter melts. Beat the eggs and add the almond milk in a separate bowl. Combine baking soda, brown rice flour and xylitol. Alternate mixing the cocoa mixture and the almond milk mixture into the dry ingredients.

Allow the batter to sit for 30 minutes before cooking. Then using a greased griddle or large frying pan on medium high, pour in 3-4 TBSP of the batter and by moving the pan, quickly spread the batter evenly to make a thin, round shape. Flip the crêpe after 1 minute or when the cooked side is slightly browned. Heat the second side for only 10 seconds. Remove from pan and place on a dish. Put wax paper between each crêpe so they do not stick together.

Filling Preparations:

Place all the filling ingredients (except the xanthan gum) in a pan on medium heat, bring to a simmer, and then slowly stir in the xanthan gum until thickened. Put a generous amount of filling down the middle of each crêpe, roll and place on a warmed plate. Keep warm until served. Serves 8-10.

Tasty Pumpkin Pie ★★★

Ingredients:

1	Unbaked, spelt pie shell	½	tsp maple flavoring
10-12 oz. silken tofu		½	tsp stevia powder
⅓	cup coconut oil	¼	tsp sea salt
1	can (15 oz.) pumpkin	1	tsp cinnamon
2	TBSP agave nectar	½	tsp ginger
1	TBSP xylitol	¼	tsp nutmeg

Preparations:

Preheat oven to 350°F. Blend all the ingredients for the filling until smooth and creamy in a blender or food processor. If using a blender, start with some of the tofu and oil. Using the pulse button; gradually add the rest of the ingredients, stirring between pulses. Pour into the unbaked pie shell. Bake for 1 hour. Chill and serve. Serves 8.

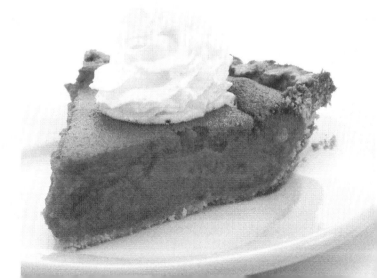

Raw Berry Pie with Almond Crust ★★★

Ingredients for Almond Pie Crust:

1 cup soaked almonds	2 TBSP tahini
⅓ cup raisins	1 tsp vanilla extract

Preparations:

Soak 1 cup of almonds in 2 cups of purified water overnight and drain. Pulse-chop all the ingredients together in a food processor. You may need to stop and scrape down the sides of the food processor, adding 1-2 TBSP of water a couple times while processing as this mixture will be thick, and may ball up in the processor. Just work it down so the ingredients are thoroughly mixed together. With wet fingers, spread the almond mixture into a 9-inch pie dish. Freeze the pie crust for 1 hour to set, or bake it at 250°F for 30 minutes and cool. Yields 1 crust.

Ingredients for Berry Filling:

1 pint strawberries, whole	1 TBSP agar-agar flakes
1 pint raspberries	3 TBSP agave nectar
1 cup fruit juice (mango, orange or raspberry)	

Preparations:

Trim and wash the strawberries and raspberries and put them on a cloth towel to drain. Arrange on the almond pie crust. Mix the fruit juice with agar-agar flakes in a small pot, bring to a boil for 1 minute, then simmer for another minute. Let stand a couple of minutes before pouring over the fruit. Place the pie in the refrigerator and allow to set for another 30 minutes. Delicious with Mango Cream (see page 180).

Banana Bread ★★★

Ingredients:

½ cup unsweetened applesauce	2 cups whole wheat flour
¼ cup coconut yogurt (So Delicious™)	½ tsp salt
1 cup mashed bananas	½ tsp baking powder
½ cup ground flax seed	½ tsp baking soda
½ cup xylitol or sucanat	

Preparations:

Cream together the applesauce, eggs, xylitol and coconut yogurt. Add the flour, salt, baking powder, baking soda, and mashed bananas. Mix until combined. Pour into bread pans and bake at 375°F for about a half hour.

Suggestion - do not make the bread too thick or it will not bake thoroughly; make the layer of dough rather thin, and it will be delicious.

Sarah's Best Banana Bread Ever ✶✶

Ingredients:

1¼ cup spelt flour	1-2 eggs
¼ cup ground flax seeds	½ cup applesauce
½ cup rolled oats	½ cup vanilla coconut yogurt (So Delicious™)
¾ cup xylitol or sucanat	1 tsp vanilla extract
1 tsp baking powder	2 medium ripe bananas
1 tsp cinnamon	½ cup walnut pieces
½ tsp nutmeg	¾ cup chocolate chips

Preparations

1. Preheat your oven to 350°F and lightly grease a loaf pan.

2. Mash the bananas and mix with the egg, yogurt, xylitol, applesauce, and vanilla extract.

3. In a separate bowl, mix the flour, flax seeds, baking powder, oats, cinnamon and nutmeg together.

4. Combine dry and wet until just mixed. Fold in the nuts and chocolate chips. Spoon the mixture into your prepared loaf pan.

5. Bake in preheated oven at 350°F oven for about 1 hour. Check to see if the loaf is ready by inserting a knife or toothpick into the center of the loaf. It should come out completely clean when it's ready.

6. Cool in the loaf pan for 10 minutes and then remove from the loaf pan and allow to cool on a wire rack.

TIPS: If your mixture looks too dry you can add a little more applesauce. Remove nuts if you are allergic. Change out walnuts for macadamia or pecans.

Sneaky Bundt Cake (Veggie Pulp!) ★

Ingredients:

2   cups mixed flour (oat and wheat)
1½ cups xylitol and or sucanat
2   TBS ground chia seed
2   tsp cinnamon
½   tsp nutmeg
½   tsp sea salt
1   tsp baking soda
1   tsp baking powder
3   eggs, beaten

1½ tsp vanilla extract
4   ripe large bananas
2   cups loosely packed veggie pulp
     (carrots, apple)
2   TBS molasses
1   cup mixed chopped nuts (walnuts,
     pumpkin seeds, or pecans)
1   cup Thompson raisins (or other
     dried fruit mix)

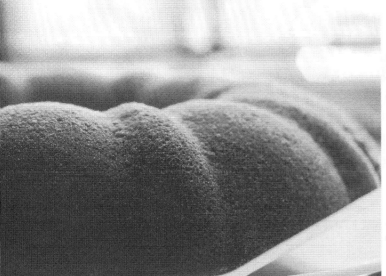

Preparation:

Pull out 2 large bowls, 1 small bowl, and 1 bundt pan. In the first bowl combine all the wet ingredients, in the second bowl combine all the dry ingredients, and in the third bowl combine the nuts and dried fruit. Add the dry ingredients to the wet and mix together. Fold in the nuts and dried fruit. Using a spatula, pour the mixture into the bunt pan. Use the spatula to flatten and even the ingredients in the mold.

Bake at 375°F for 50 minutes. Allow to cool before removing the cake from the pan. Serves 12.

Fudge Black Bean Brownies ★★★

Note: Yes, these taste great! Try them for yourself. If you cook the black beans, make sure you do not add anything other than sea salt to them. To save money, make your own black beans for use in the recipe.

Ingredients:

15½-oz. can black beans, drained and
     rinsed very well
3   large eggs
3   TBSP coconut oil (melted to liquid)
¾   cup xylitol or granulated sugar
½   cup cocoa powder

1   tsp vanilla extract
½   tsp peppermint extract, optional
½   tsp baking powder
Pinch salt
½   cup mini chocolate chips, divided

Preparations:

1. Preheat the oven to 350°F. Spray an 8 x 8-inch baking pan with nonstick cooking spray and set aside.

2. Place the black beans in the bowl of a food processor; process until smooth and creamy. Add the eggs, oil, sugar, cocoa powder, vanilla extract, peppermint extract, baking powder, and salt and process until smooth. Add ¼ cup of the chips and pulse a few times until the chips are broken up a bit.

3. Pour batter into the prepared baking dish and sprinkle the top with the remaining ¼ cup chocolate chips.

4. Bake 30 to 35 minutes, or until the edges start to pull away from the sides and a toothpick inserted in the center comes out clean. Cool in the pan before slicing. Makes 16 servings.

Vegan Pecan Pie **

Ingredients:

1	cup brown rice syrup	2	TBSP spelt flour
½	cup chia gel (1 part chia to 4 parts water)	1	tsp vanilla
		1	cup chopped pecans
¾	cup sucanat	1	cup whole pecans
2	TBSP molasses	1	9" unbaked pastry crust
¼	tsp salt		

Preparations:

Preheat the oven to 350°F. Vigorously beat together the brown rice syrup, chia gel, sucanat, molasses, salt, flour, and whisk in the vanilla using a spoon. Fold in the chopped pecans and whole pecans. Pour filling into 9" pie crust.

Bake on the center rack of oven for 65-70 minutes. Cool for 2 hours on wire rack before serving. Serves 8.

Tip: Tapping the center surface of pie lightly will not work with this recipe, as there are no eggs. You will notice that it will be almost done when the amount of bubbling is reduced by half. Do not cook longer than 75 minutes.

Vegan Pumpkin Pie – No Tofu ★★★★

Note: MAKE THIS THE DAY BEFORE SERVING. It needs a day to set before eating. Also note that this filling is spicy.

Ingredients:

2 cups solid-pack canned pumpkin	1 tsp ground cinnamon
1 cup coconut milk	1 tsp vanilla
¾ cup sucanat	½ tsp EACH ground ginger, nutmeg and salt
2 TBSP ground chia seed	¼ tsp ground allspice or cloves
1 TBSP blackstrap molasses	1 9" unbaked pastry crust

Preparations:

Preheat oven to 350°F. Blend all the ingredients, except the pie crust, in the blender, for 20 seconds, or until it creamy and without chunks. Pour the filling in the center of the pie pastry, using a spatula to scrape out any batter remaining in the blender.

Bake the pie for 60 minutes. Cool on a rack, then refrigerate overnight before serving. Serves 8.

Chia Energy Cookies ★★

Ingredients:

½ cup + 1 TBSP coconut oil	1 cup spelt flour
4 TBSP cocoa	1 tsp baking soda
⅛ tsp cinnamon	Dash salt
¾ cup xylitol	2 TBSP chia seeds
1 egg	½ cup chocolate chips
1 tsp vanilla	1 cup chopped walnuts

Preparations:

Drop cookies by teaspoonful on a parchment paper covered cookie sheet. Bake at 325°F for 10-12 minutes. The cookies do not spread out. They keep nicely for a week.

Two cookies provide energy (without sugar lows) for about three hours.

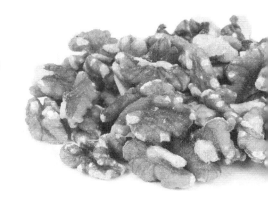

Mango Cream ★★★★

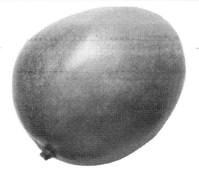

Ingredients:

8 oz. mango chunks
5 TBSP coconut milk
sweetener to taste

Preparations:

Pulse-chop mangos in your food processor with 2 TBSP coconut (or almond) milk and your pre-ferred sweetener (if desired). When softened, add the rest of the milk and purée until creamy.

Store in freezer or serve immediately. Serves 2.

Chocolate Cashew Butter Cups ★★

Ingredients:

1 cup cashew or almond butter
¼ tsp sea salt

½ cup xylitol (Emerald Forest™)
12 oz. bittersweet chocolate chips

Preparations:

Place the nut butter in a jar or bowl and set over boiling water until the butter gets soft. In a small bowl, mix the nut butter, sea salt, and xylitol until firm. Place this mix to the side, covering with a towel to keep warm.

Melt the chocolate chips in a double boiler over hot, but not boiling, water. Grease muffin tin cups or use paper liners. Spoon some chocolate into each cup, filling halfway. Then, with the smooth side of the spoon, draw the chocolate up the edges of each cup until all sides are coated. Place this into the refrigerator and cool for 2 minutes. Spread about ½ tsp of the nut butter mix into each chocolate-lined cup. Pour some chocolate onto the top of each candy and spread it to the edges. Garnish the butter cups with crushed nuts. Cover with a towel and place in the refrigerator until firm. Turn out of the pan when done.

Store them in the refrigerator or in a cool spot. Yields 8-10 candies.

Chocolate Chip Cookies **

Tip: Tahini is sesame butter available at health food stores.

Ingredients:

¼ cup tahini
¼ cup water
⅓ cup spelt flour
⅓ cup applesauce
½ cup granola of choice

1 tsp vanilla extract
½ cup granola (yes another cup)
½ cup walnuts, finely chopped
½ cup chocolate or carob chips

Preparations:

Preheat oven to 350°F. Put the tahini, water, spelt flour, applesauce, ½ cup granola, and vanilla in the food processor and blend for a few seconds until creamy. Scrape mixture into a medium bowl. Stir in the remaining ½ cup granola, walnuts, and chocolate chips. Drop the cookie dough by tablespoonfuls onto a greased baking sheet and press down.

Bake for 18 minutes. Yields 10-12 cookies.

Oatmeal Cookies **

Ingredients:

½ cup butter or sunflower oil
1 cup xylitol (Emerald Forest™)
1 egg
⅓ cup coconut or hemp milk
½ tsp vanilla extract
1½ cups spelt flour
½ tsp baking soda

½ tsp sea salt (Redmond's RealSalt™)
1 tsp cinnamon
2½ cups rolled oats
¾ cup raisins, chocolate chips, or carob chips (optional)
½ cup chopped walnuts (optional)

Preparations:

Preheat oven to 350°F. Cream together the sugar, vanilla, and butter or oil in a medium mixing bowl. Add the egg and coconut milk and beat until well mixed. Add the vanilla extract.

In a separate bowl, sift together the flour, soda, salt, and cinnamon. Gradually add this to the sugar mixture, mixing well. Then stir in the rolled oats, raisins, chocolate chips, and walnuts.

Drop the cookie dough by tablespoonfuls onto a greased baking sheet and press down. Bake for 10-12 minutes. Yields 10-12 cookies.

Cashew Whipped Cream ★★★

Ingredients:

1 cup almonds or cashews	1 TBSP maple syrup (optional)
¾ cup water	½ tsp vanilla extract (optional)

Preparations:

Soak 1 cup of almonds or cashews in 2 cups of water overnight. If you're in a warm climate, soak them in your refrigerator. After 8-12 hours, drain the soaking water and rinse the nuts. In a blender, place the nuts and enough fresh water to allow the blade to operate. Blend gradually, adding water to achieve a smooth consistency. Add maple syrup and vanilla if desired. Yields 1 ½ cups.

Lemon Crème ★

Tip: This is a creamy whipped topping, delicious over any pie, cake, fruit cup or chilled fruit soup.

Ingredients:

10 oz. silken tofu	2 TBSP maple syrup (Shady Maple™)
2 TBSP tofu mayonnaise	or stevia (KAL™ or Sweet Leaf™)
4 TBSP pineapple juice concentrate	to taste
5 TBSP lime juice	

Preparations:

Place all ingredients into a blender or a food processor and process until creamy smooth. Then refrigerate to chill. Yields enough for 1 pie.

Dairy-Free Chocolate Pudding Recipe ★★

Ingredients:

2 cup sliced bananas	1 tsp vanilla extract
¼ cup coconut milk (organic)	½ tsp nutmeg
¼ cup almond flour	½ tsp sea salt
1 tsp almond extract	½ cup chia gel (1 part chia to 4 parts water)
1 cup semi-sweet dark chocolate chips	

Preparations:

Pour half of the coconut milk into a blender. Add one or two slices of banana and blend. Keep adding banana one slice at a time until they are all blended, adding the rest of the coconut milk as needed so it will blend. Add chocolate chips, sea salt, vanilla extract, almond extract, nutmeg, almond flour, and blend. Once you've got everything else blended, add the chia gel and blend. You'll see that it disappears right into the mix and you won't even know it's there except for the fact that it adds a nice, thick consistency.

Pour pudding into bowls and chill in refrigerator for several hours. I like to serve mine in small Japanese teacups, which are perfect for individual servings. Yields 3 cups or 24 ounces of pudding.

Fudge Drops *

Ingredients:

- ¼ cup agave nectar or honey
- 3   TBSP sunflower oil
- 3   TBSP apple juice
- 1   tsp vanilla extract
- 1   cup spelt flour

- ⅓ cup raw or toasted carob powder
- 1   tsp cream of tartar
- ½ TBSP baking soda
- ⅓ cup chopped cashews

Preparations:

Preheat oven to 325°F. Combine the honey, oil, and apple juice in a medium saucepan. Briefly heat to melt the honey, then remove from heat and stir in the vanilla.

In a separate bowl sift together the flour, carob powder, cream of tartar, and baking soda. Stir the wet ingredients slowly into the flour mixture, and then stir in the nuts. Drop rounded teaspoonfuls onto a greased cookie sheet.

Bake for 15-18 minutes. Yields 8-10 drops.

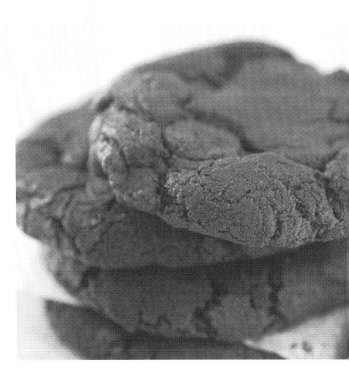

Creamy Carrot Cake ★★

Ingredients:

1¾ cup spelt flour or brown rice flour	1 cup raisins
2 tsp baking soda	½ cup coconut, shredded
2 tsp cinnamon	3 eggs
½ tsp nutmeg	¾ cup honey
¼ tsp cloves	½ cup sunflower oil
2 dashes stevia (KAL™ or Sweet Leaf™)	½ cup walnuts, chopped
2½ cups carrots, grated	1 **Creamy Maple Frosting Recipe** (below)
8 oz. pineapple, crushed with liquids	

Preparations:

Preheat oven to 325°F. Sift the flour, baking soda, cinnamon, nutmeg, cloves, and stevia into a bowl. Resift and set aside. In a large bowl, combine the carrots, pineapple, raisins, and coconut. Set aside.

In a medium mixing bowl, beat the eggs. Add the honey in a thin stream while beating until the mixture is light and frothy. Continue beating while adding the oil. Pour the egg mixture into the carrot mixture. Stir gently to combine. Sift half of the flour mixture over the bowl and gently fold in. Repeat with the remaining flour. Fold in the walnuts. Pour into a greased 7½" x 11¾" baking pan or in two 8" or 9" round cake pans (for a double-layered carrot cake).

Bake for 50 minutes (for the large pan) or 35-40 minutes (for the round pans). Allow to cool in pans for 10 minutes, then carefully turn out onto wire racks and finish cooling. Frost with Creamy Maple Frosting. Serves 10-15.

Creamy Maple Frosting ★★★

Ingredients:

1 12 oz. pkg. silken tofu	1 tsp vanilla extract
½ cup raw cashews (or other nuts)	½ tsp cinnamon
3 TBSP maple syrup (Shady Maple™)	Pinch sea salt
3 TBSP sucanat	

Preparations:

Cut tofu into slices. Place into a steamer basket in a medium saucepan and steam for 5 minutes. Drain tofu between several layers of cloth towels for at least 10 minutes.

Blend cashews, maple syrup, sucanat, vanilla, sea salt, and cinnamon until smooth. Add the tofu a little at a time, blending until the mixture is smooth and creamy. Scrape the sides of the container as needed.

Chill before spreading on cake. Makes enough frosting for one cake.

Toasted Coconut Ice Cream **

Ingredients:

1   cup unsweetened coconut, shredded
4   cups unsweetened coconut milk
    (So Delicious™)
2   tsp cornstarch

1   cup xylitol (Emerald Forest™)
1   large egg
1   large egg white

Preparations:

Preheat oven to 325° F. Spread the coconut in a thin layer on a rimmed baking sheet and toast in the middle of the oven, stirring frequently, until lightly golden, about 5 minutes. Set aside to cool. Whisk the milk and cornstarch in a large saucepan until blended. Add the xylitol and eggs, and cook over medium-low heat, whisking constantly, until the xylitol is dissolved and the mixture is slightly thickened, about 8 minutes. Do not boil this mixture! Remove from heat and allow the custard to cool slightly.

Whisk the coconut milk and toasted coconut into the custard until well blended. Transfer the mixture to a large metal bowl. Set the bowl in a basin of ice water and let stand until cooled to room temperature. Stir mixture occasionally.

Cover and place in freezer for at least 6 hours or overnight, to allow the flavors to fully mingle. Then process the custard in an ice cream maker according to the manufacturer's directions. Turn into a bowl with a tight-fitting lid. Place a piece of plastic wrap directly on top of the ice cream before storing in freezer. Serves 5.

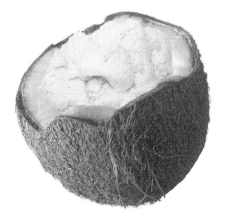

SAUCES, DIPS, SPREADS & SALAD DRESSINGS

Recipes that repair your health!

The recipes, for some of the dressings, are left with an open amount for the spices so you can add more or less according to your taste. Use these sauces for salad dressings, dips, and spreads. If you want to reduce the overall calorie and sugar amount, substitute the honey or agave nectar with stevia. Substitute ½ cup applesauce per ¼ cup oil. If you are unsure what some of the ingredients are refer to the Food Beautiful Shopping List or the Fabulous Food Replacement Section.

Kickin' Garlic Dressing ★★★★

Ingredients:

½ cup coconut oil	⅓ cup liquid aminos (Bragg™)
2 tsp lemon pepper blend	¼ cup apple cider vinegar
2 tsp basil	¼ cup agave nectar or raw honey
1 tsp thyme	¼ tsp sea salt
6 cloves garlic, minced	

Preparation:

Turn stove top burner onto medium high, place the coconut oil into sauce pan allow to warm up. Add lemon pepper, basil, and thyme to the oil, and allow to simmer for 2 minutes. Turn down the heat if
necessary--don't burn the oil. After about 2 minutes remove oil from heat and add the minced garlic, then the liquid aminos, apple cider vinegar, and agave, and mix together. Poor into an empty glass jar and serve on salad or toast. This salad dressing does not require refrigeration. Yields 1½ cups.

Lavender-Lemon Cream ★★

Ingredients:

½ cup silken tofu or cream	2 tsp lavender buds
½ cup rice or tofu cream cheese	¼ tsp sea salt (Redmond's RealSalt™)
2 TBSP agave nectar	zest of 1 lemon

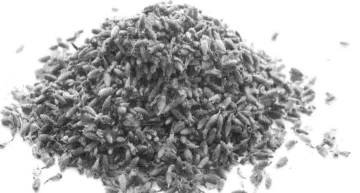

Preparations:

Beat the silken tofu and rice cream cheese together. Heat agave nectar in a small pan on low, allowing it to melt, then add the lavender buds and stir until coated. Remove from the heat and press the buds with a spoon until finely mixed. Fold the lavender mixture into the cream mixture and add the zest of 1 lemon. Allow to sit for a couple hours to pull out the oils. Spread on sprouted bagels!

To use as a sauce, add ¼ cup water and mix together on medium low heat. Serve with lamb or chicken. Yields 2 cups.

Royal Flavor ★★★★

Ingredients:

½   cup tahini
¼   cup lemon juice
¼   cup rice milk or water
1   TBSP poppy seeds
½   tsp red pepper flakes

½   tsp ground white pepper
¼   cup parsley or cilantro, finely chopped
1   tsp sea salt (Redmond's RealSalt™)
2   dashes powdered stevia (KAL™ or Sweet Leaf™)

Preparations:

Mix all ingredients in a pan on medium heat until creamy. Serve with Roasted Vegetables. Yields 1¼ cups.

Sweet & Sour Pineapple Sauce ★★★

Ingredients:

¼   cup pineapple chunks with half the juice
2   TBSP fruit-sweetened ketchup (Muir Glen Organics™)
2   TBSP red wine or sherry
1   tsp cornstarch
2   TBSP paprika
2   TBSP liquid aminos (Bragg™)
4   TBSP sunflower oil

Preparations:

Mix all ingredients in a pan on medium heat until slightly thick. Serve over meat and vegetables. Yields 1½ cups.

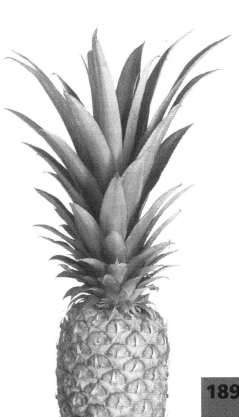

Strawberry Sweet ★★★

Ingredients:

1   cup fresh strawberries
¼   cup sunflower oil

½   tsp sea salt (Redmond RealSalt™)
2   TBSP maple syrup (Shady Maple™)

Preparations:

Blend together until smooth. Toss with greens and add fresh strawberries, walnuts, and raw, sharp cheddar cheese. Yields ¾ cup.

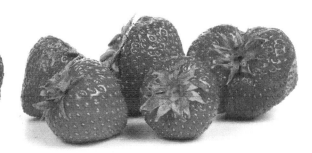

Tahini Mint ★★★★

Ingredients:

2   TBSP tahini (sesame butter)
2   cloves garlic, pressed
1   TBSP dried mint
½   cup pure water

1   TBSP lemon or lime juice
1   tsp white miso (optional)
1   TBSP apple cider vinegar (Bragg™)
¼   cup sesame oil

Preparations:

Blend until smooth and chill. Yields 1½ cup.

Curried Dressing ★★★★

Ingredients

½   cup sunflower seeds
1   cup water
1   lemon, peeled
1   tsp sea salt (Redmond's RealSalt™)
1   tsp curry paste

½   TBSP bouillon
3   dashes cayenne
½   tsp cumin
1   cup tomato juice blend
½   green onion, chopped

Preparations:

Soak sunflower seeds in water overnight. Drain. Blend with 1 cup water until smooth. Add peeled lemon, along with remaining ingredients. Blend well. Serve hot or cold over roasted or steamed vegetables. Yields 1¼ cups.

Creamy Ranchero ★★★★

Ingredients

10 oz. silken tofu
¼ cup onion, chopped
1 clove garlic, minced or pressed
1 tsp liquid aminos (Bragg™)
1 tsp cumin

½ tsp dill weed
2 TBSP lemon juice
2 TBSP vegan mayonnaise (Follow Your Heart™)

Preparations:

Blend until creamy and chill. Yields 2 cups.

Chile Ginger Sauce ★★★★

Ingredients

4 red chiles (pulp, no skin)
½ tsp cumin
1 TBSP garlic, minced
¾ cup water
½ TBSP liquid aminos (Bragg™)

1 TBSP ginger, juiced or grated
10½ oz. silken tofu
½ tsp honey or stevia (KAL™ or Sweet Leaf™) to taste
1 TBSP orange juice

Preparations:

Blend until creamy. Heat on low in small saucepan and serve warm. Use for an Asian coleslaw sauce or on salads. Yields 1 cup.

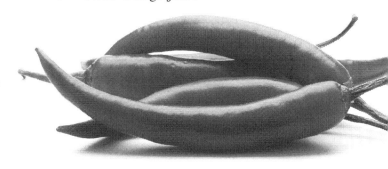

Ginger Cashew Sauce ★★★

Ingredients

2 TBSP cashew butter
3 TBSP lemon juice
1 TBSP liquid aminos or tamari
1½ TBSP fresh ginger, skinned and chopped

¼ tsp hot pepper sauce or cayenne to taste
1 TBSP toasted sesame oil
3 tsp honey or liquid stevia, to taste

Preparations:

Blend until smooth and creamy. Serve this on Asian salads or noodles. Yields ¾ cup.

Red Roque Vinaigrette ✶✶✶✶

Ingredients

1   cup fresh tomatoes, chopped
2   TBSP nutritional yeast flakes
¾   cup water
3   TBSP olive oil
½   tsp sea salt (Redmond's RealSalt™)
½   tsp thyme

½   tsp dill weed
2   cloves garlic, minced or pressed
½   tsp white pepper
3   dashes powdered stevia (KAL™ or Sweet Leaf™)

Preparations:

Blend all ingredients until smooth and creamy. Keep leftovers bottled in fridge. Great with leafy greens and pasta salads. Yields 2 cups.

Avocado Lime Sauce ✶✶✶✶

Ingredients

⅓   cup avocado, mashed
2   TBSP apple cider vinegar (Bragg™)
½   cup lime juice
2   cloves garlic, minced or pressed
1   serrano chile, seeded and chopped (optional)
3   TBSP vegan mayonnaise (Follow Your Heart™)
½   cup water
sea salt and white pepper to taste
2   dashes stevia (KAL™ or Sweet Leaf™)

Preparations:

Blend until smooth. Yields 1½ cups.

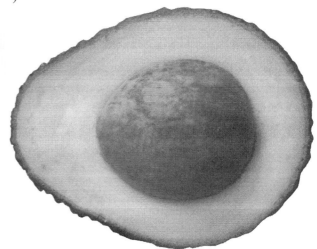

Sweet Tomato Vinaigrette ✱✱✱

Ingredients

1   tsp fruit-sweetened ketchup
    (Muir Glen Organics™)
1   tsp liquid aminos (Bragg™)
2   tsp olive oil
¼   cup brown rice vinegar

½   TBSP roasted red pepper sauce
2   tsp honey or use stevia (KAL™ or
    Sweet Leaf™) to taste
1   cup tomato, seeded and finely chopped
1   TBSP parsley, minced

Preparations:

Whisk together the first six ingredients, then stir in tomato and parsley. Chill and serve.
Yields 1½ cups.

Cucumber Dressing ✱✱✱

Ingredients

½   cup cucumber, skinned, seeded
    and chopped
2   TBSP sunflower oil
½   TBSP liquid aminos (Bragg™) or
    soy sauce

½   cup vegan mayonnaise (Follow
    Your Heart™)
4   dill pickles
2   TBSP pickle juice
2   TBSP lemon juice

Preparations:

Blend until creamy. Yields 1¼ cups.

Papaya Lime Dressing ✱✱✱

Ingredients

1   cup ripe papaya (½ papaya)
2½   TBSP lime juice
1   tsp dijon mustard
½   tsp cracked white pepper

⅛   tsp sea salt (Redmond's RealSalt™)
2   TBSP water
2   TBSP agave nectar or stevia (KAL™ or
     Sweet Leaf™) to taste

Preparations:

Cut papaya, scoop out seeds, peel skin, and chop. Blend all ingredients until creamy.
Yields 1⅓ cups.

Fresh From The Garden ★★★★

Ingredients

1 cup plain goat yogurt or kefir	1 tsp thyme
¼ cup lemon juice	1 tsp oregano
¼ cup olive oil or sesame oil	4 TBSP agave nectar (to taste)
1 tsp basil	1 tsp sea salt (Redmond's RealSalt™)

Preparations:

Blend until smooth and chill. Yields 1¾ cups.

Cole Slaw Dressing ★★★

Ingredients

½ cup vegan mayonnaise (Follow Your Heart™)	2 TBSP poppy seeds
3 TBSP orange juice	1 dash cinnamon
¼ cup olive oil or sesame oil	1 tsp sea salt (Redmond's RealSalt™)
2 dashes cayenne pepper	½ cup honey or stevia (KAL™ or Sweet Leaf™) powder (to taste)
2 TBSP orange oil	

Preparations:

Blend until smooth and chill. Yields 1¼ cups.

Veggie Ranch Dip ★★★★

Ingredients

2 cups tofu sour cream (Tofutti™)	½ tsp sea salt (Redmond's RealSalt™)
2 tsp worcestershire sauce	1 tsp dill weed
¼ cup horseradish	½ tsp paprika
1 tsp celery seed, crushed	½ cup black olives, chopped

Preparations:

Combine all ingredients until well mixed. Place in refrigerator for 30 minutes to draw out the flavors. Yields 3 cups.

No Cheese Cheesy Dippin' Sauce ★★★

Ingredients:

3	cups water	2	TBSP onion, minced
½	cup rolled oats	½	TBSP tamari or liquid aminos (Bragg™)
½	cup nutritional yeast flakes	1	tsp basil
¼	cup tahini	½	tsp thyme
¼	cup arrowroot powder	3	dashes cayenne
2	TBSP lemon juice	1	clove garlic, minced or pressed
⅛	tsp turmeric powder		

Preparations:

Blend all ingredients until smooth. Pour into a small saucepan and heat to a boil, stirring constantly with a whisk until thickened. Yields 4 cups.

Lemon Balm & Hyssop Fusion ★★★★

Ingredients:

3	TBSP fresh cilantro	¼	tsp xanthan gum
1	tsp lemon grass	2	tsp liquid aminos (Bragg™)
1	tsp hyssop or fresh thyme	1	TBSP dried red bell peppers
1	tsp basil	3	TBSP mango juice
⅛	tsp paprika	¼	cup kefir or plain yogurt
⅛	tsp cinnamon		

Preparations:

Mix all ingredients, except the xanthan gum, in a food processor for 3 minutes. While blade is still turning add the xanthan gum. Chill and serve. Tastes great on salads or steamed vegetables, especially zucchini, sautéed onion, and broccoli. Yields 1¼ cups.

Ginger Cashew Pesto ★★★★

Ingredients:

½   cup raw cashews
1   cup cilantro leaves
3   TBSP lime juice
3   TBSP honey
¼   cup toasted sesame oil

2   cloves garlic, minced or pressed
2   tsp ginger root peeled and minced
1-2 dashes cayenne
1   tsp sea salt (Redmond's RealSalt™)
1   tsp paprika

Preparations:

Place all ingredients in a blender or food processor, and using the "S" blade, pulse chop to slightly chunky. Place in refrigerator and chill until served.

Spread this pesto over a spelt pizza crust, top with 2 cups grated zucchini and 1½ cups grated goat cheese or mozzarella rice cheese, and bake at 425°F for 10-12 minutes. Yields 1½ cups pesto.

Fire Roasted Hummus ★★★★

Tip: Turn this into raw hummus by soaking 2 cups of dry garbanzo beans in water for 24 hours. Drain beans and use instead of the canned beans.

Ingredients:

14 oz. garbanzo beans
5   TBSP tahini
3   cloves garlic, minced or pressed
zest of ½ lemon
juice of 1 lemon
2   pinches cayenne pepper
½   cup olive oil

1½ tsp sea salt (Redmond's RealSalt™)
2   fire roasted red peppers
¼   tsp white pepper
2   TBSP paprika
3   dashes stevia powder
¼   tsp ground cumin

Preparations:

Using a food processor or blender, purée the garbanzo beans, roasted red pepper, lemon zest, and olive oil until smooth. Add tahini, garlic, lemon juice, paprika, cayenne, cumin, sea salt, pepper and stevia (to taste). Add 2-3 TBSP of water if too thick.

Serve with warmed, sprouted grain pita bread, baby carrots, or chips. Yields 2½ cups.

Thai Red Curry Sauce ★★★★

Ingredients:

2   cloves garlic, minced or pressed
2   roasted red bell peppers, chopped
1   TBSP ginger root, chopped or pressed
2   TBSP fresh mint, roughly chopped
¼   onion, chopped
¾   cup lime juice
1   tsp ground cumin

2-3 pinches ground cloves
cayenne pepper, to taste
¾   tsp paprika
14 oz. coconut milk (Nature's Forest™)
2   TBSP red curry
½   cup xylitol (Emerald Forest™)

Preparations:

In a food processor or blender process the garlic, roasted bell peppers, ginger, mint, onion, lime juice, cayenne, cumin, cloves and paprika. Set aside. In a large saucepan simmer the coconut milk, then add the red curry sauce and xylitol and stir for 5 minutes.

Pour over a bed of brown rice topped with steamed broccoli, cabbage, carrots, and baby corn. You can also serve with white fish or other organic white meat. Yields 3½ cups.

Green Curry Sauce ★★★★

Ingredients:

4   cloves garlic, minced or pressed
2-3 mild chilies, chopped
1   TBSP ginger root, chopped or pressed
2   dashes cayenne pepper
1   tsp ground cumin
2-3 pinches ground cloves
1   pinch cinnamon

¼   onion, chopped
½   cup lemon juice
14 oz. coconut milk (Nature's Forest™)
2   TBSP green curry
½   cup honey
1   TBSP liquid aminos (Bragg™)

Preparations:

In a food processor or blender process the garlic, ginger, chilies, onion, lemon juice, cayenne, cumin, cloves, and cinnamon. Set aside. In a large saucepan simmer the coconut milk, and then add the green curry sauce and honey. Stir occasionally for 5 minutes.

Best served hot over vegetables or for dipping! Yields 3½ cups.

Reminiscent Peanut Sauce ★★★

Avoid peanuts! Many fungi naturally produce a substance known as a mycotoxin during their digestive process. These mycotoxins are toxic to humans, and some are extremely toxic if ingested even in small quantities. One study found as many as 24 different forms of fungi in peanuts alone. The one thing worth mentioning here is that there is no good way to even begin to eliminate these fungi and mycotoxins from shell nuts.

Ingredients:

½ cup almond butter
2   TBSP lemon juice
1   TBSP fresh ginger, minced
2   TBSP maple syrup or raw agave nectar
1   TBSP tamari or liquid aminos (Bragg™)

2   cloves garlic, minced
1   tsp Thai red chili paste
½   tsp sea salt, or to taste
¼   tsp white or black pepper
¼   cup water

Preparations:

Blend all ingredients until smooth. Yields 1 cup.

RECIPES FOR JUICING

Before you juice, wash the vegetables thoroughly and cut them into small enough pieces to fit through the mouth of the juicer. It is recommended that you dilute the juice by 1/3 water as the virgin juice can be too concentrated for the stomach. For example, if you have 12 ounces of fresh juice, add 4 ounces of water.

It is suggested on the first two sips to swish the juice around in your mouth for 15 seconds to activate your digestive enzymes. This can prevent the stomach from experiencing any stress. Juice helps in the absorption and utilization of calcium supplements, cod liver oil and multivitamins, so they can be taken together.

Each juice recipe yields about 12-16 ounces of juice. You can save time juicing every day by making 1 large batch and freezing the juice in glass jars. Make sure to dilute the juice and leave about 1 inch space between the juice and the lid, so the glass doesn't break. Enjoy the recipes and feel free to create your own wonderful juices!

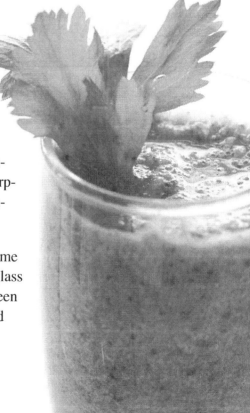

Green Machine ★★★★

½ bunch of spinach
1 large handful parsley
2 stalks celery
1 apple
4 carrots

The Real V8 Juice ★★★★

2 tomatoes
2 stalks celery
1 clove garlic
¼ yellow onion
2 handfuls parsley or cilantro

Ginger With Greens ★★★★

½ cucumber
½ bunch of spinach
2 stalks celery
1" slice of fresh ginger
1 apple

A Full Salad ★★★★

1 tomato
6 romaine lettuce leaves
2 stalks celery
2 carrots
2 handfuls spinach
¼ onion
1 clove garlic

Color Me A Rainbow ★★★★

½ beet
1 apple
2 stalks celery
3 carrots
1 handful parsley
2 cups red cabbage

Carrot Lemon Juice ★★★★

4 carrots
3 stalks celery
½ lemon
1 apple
½ bunch of spinach

Sweet As Ever ★★★★

1 apple
5 carrots
3 stalks celery
1 orange, peeled

Beet Sweet ★★★★

½ beet, with top
1 apple
2 stalks celery

Clean As A Whistle ★★★★

4 carrots
½ head spinach
1 handful parsley
½ onion
1 clove garlic
1 apple

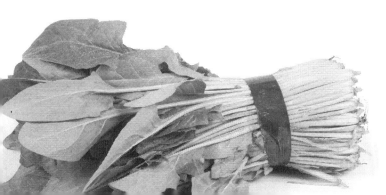

Broccoli & Carrot ★★★★

1-2 broccoli spears
3 carrots
1 grapefruit, without peel
1 apple
1 handful parsley
3 stalks celery

Tummy Tonic ★★★★

¼ inch slice of ginger
½ cup peppermint or spearmint leaves
½ pineapple with skin

Oh So Green ★★★★

4 stalks celery
½ cucumber
1 handful of spinach
1 handful of parsley
1 apple

Fruits For Immune Power ★★★★

Zest from ⅛ of the orange
1 orange, peeled
½ pineapple with skin
½ cup strawberries
1 banana, peeled

Juice the first 4 ingredients, then blend the juice and banana until liquefied.

Mexicali Juice ★★★★

1 jicama
4 carrots
1 apple
2 stalks celery

Purple Delight ★★★★

½ head red cabbage
3 carrots
½ lime
2 stalks celery

Body Cooler ★★★★

1 tomato or apple
1 cucumber
3 stalks celery
½ cup peppermint (optional)

Immuno-power ★★★★

1 cup Jerusalem artichoke
2 carrots
1 handful of parsley
2 cloves garlic
¼ inch slice ginger
1 apple

Fennel Tummy Tonic ★★★★

1 handful peppermint or spearmint
1 rib of fennel
2 apples

Melon Aid ★★

½ cantaloupe
Zest from ¼ lemon
½ lemon
1 apple
1 kiwi

You can substitute any melon of choice.

Fruit Potassium Punch ★★★★

1 peach, pitted
½ papaya
2 oranges, peeled
1 banana

Juice first 3 ingredients, then blend juice and banana until liquefied.

Kidney Tonic ★★★★

Zest of ¼ lemon
½ lemon
20 grapes
1 cup cranberries
2 apples

Ulcer Tonic ★★★★

¼ head of cabbage
1 apple
2 oz. Pure aloe vera gel
1 banana

Juice first 2 items, then use a blender to mix the veggie juice, aloe vera gel, and banana.

Veggie Potassium ★★★★

1 handful parsley
3 carrots
3 stalks celery
1 handful spinach
1 tomato

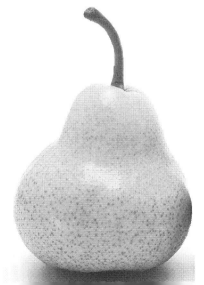

Liver Tonic ★★★★

6 dandelion leaves
½ beet with top
1 apple
3 carrots

Gallbladder Tonic ★★★★

5 radishes
1 pear
1 apple
½ beet
½ parsnip
½ lemon

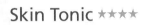

Skin Tonic ★★★★

1 apple
¼ head of cabbage
2 stalks celery
1 handful parsley

Cleansing Cocktail ★★★★

1 apple
4 carrots
½ beet
2 stalks celery

Beautiful Skin ★★★★

1 pear
2 celery stocks
¼ cup red cabbage
2 carrots

Ginger Ale ★★★★

1 lemon wedge with peel
¼ inch of ginger, pressed
1 green apple
5 oz. ginger ale (Ginger People™)

Juice first 3 ingredients, then
add the ginger ale.

Ginger-Pineapple ★★★★

½ pineapple
¼ inch of ginger
1 cup parsley or wheatgrass

MEDICINAL RECIPES FOR VARIOUS AILMENTS

Anti-Plague Tonic

Ingredients:

1   quart apple cider vinegar, raw, unfiltered, unbleached, non-distilled (Bragg™)
1   part fresh garlic cloves, minced
1   part fresh white onion, chopped (or hottest onions)
1   part fresh ginger root, finely grated
1   partfresh horseradish root, finely grated
1   part fresh chopped cayenne peppers or the hottest
     peppers available (Habanero, African Bird, or Scotch Bonnets)

Note: This formula is a modern-day plague tonic that is adapted from Dr. Christopher's original anti-plague tonic. This formula is not just for mild illnesses; it has helped to heal some of the deadliest infections like some of the new mutated killer viruses that defy conventional antibiotics. It has been said the tonic becomes even more potent when you start a batch on the new moon and end it on the new moon. This tonic is extremely powerful because all the ingredients are fresh. When this tonic is used in conjunction with a vibrant routine it can remedy the most chronic conditions and stubborn diseases. This tonic stimulates maximum blood circulation, while positioning the best detoxifying herbs into the bloodstream to kill unfamiliar agents on contact.

It can be used during pregnancies and is safe for children (for children use half the dosage, toddlers one-fourth, and infants should receive it through the mother's milk).

This is a food and is completely non-toxic. Make up plenty as it does NOT need refrigeration and lasts indefinitely without any special storage conditions.

Caution: If you plan to grind the horseradish, make sure you wear eye protection, as the volatile oils enter the air. Use the proper amounts and recommended brands for purity and efficacy. Remember that all the herbs and vegetables should be fresh (and organically-grown if possible). Use dried herbs only in an emergency.

Preparations:

1. Fill a glass jar ¾ full with equal parts (i.e. a cupful each) of the fresh chopped and grated herbs.

2. Fill the jar to the top with RAW, unfiltered, unbleached, non-dist illed apple cider vinegar. Close and shake vigorously and then top off the vinegar if necessary.

3. Shake at least once a day for two to four weeks, and then filter the mixture through a clean piece of cheese cloth or a clean unbleached white T-shirt, bottle and label. Note that it is very important to remember shaking the mixture every day or even every time you walk by it.

DOSAGE:
The dosage is ½ to 1 ounce (1-2 TBSP), two or more times daily. Gargle and swallow. DO NOT DILUTE WITH WATER.

You want the best quality items available. Before you start, stock up on organic gourmet garlic that is more powerful than conventional garlic and has over 200 medicinal compounds. To order, visit **www.charliesgourmetgarlic.com**

Joint-Ligament-Muscle Tonic

Ingredients:

2   eggs with only 1 egg yolk
2   tsp apple cider vinegar
2   tsp cod liver oil (Carlson®)
1   tsp ginger--add to recipe if problem is in the lower half of body
1   clove minced garlic--add to recipe if you have circulatory problems

Preparations:

You can first test to see if your raw eggs are safe to eat. Fill a clear glass three-fourths with water. Gently drop an egg into the water using a spoon. If the egg floats to the top throw it away, if it sinks to the bottom it is safe to eat. If you are still hesitant about eating raw eggs, combine them with garlic to kill any bacteria.

Place all ingredients in a glass cup or small jar. Using a fork, thoroughly mix together. Allow to activate for 5-10 minutes. Drink quickly.

Tummy Tonic - Crystallized Ginger Slices

Tip: Use for nausea, sea sickness, upset stomach, indigestion, and great to nibble on during pregnancy and for elderly persons who experience low appetite.

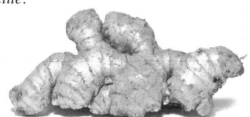

1   cup peeled, thinly sliced ginger
3   cups water
1   cup xylitol or raw sugar cane
additional sugar cane to coat (optional)

Preparations:

In a covered saucepan, bring the water to a boil. Add the ginger pieces and xylitol and cover. Reduce heat to medium low and simmer for 5 minutes. Remove from heat let mixture to sit for 20 minutes. Although you don't need the ginger water any more, you can keep it to make homemade ginger ale.

Heat the oven to 200°F. Place the ginger slices in a glass pan. Place the pan in the oven until the slices are almost dry but still chewy. Allow ginger to cool, then toss in xylitol or raw cane sugar to lightly coat it, if desired. Store the crystallized ginger in an airtight container for up to two months.

Variation:

If you do not want to use sugar in this recipe, you can make it plain, or substitute the sugar with maple syrup or raw honey, using half the amount called for in the recipe. Boil the ginger the same as directed. Instead of tossing the cooled ginger in sugar to lightly coat it, sprinkle stevia or another sugar substitute over the ginger pieces to taste.

Effective Infant Formula Recipe

Note: All of these products can be purchased at your health food store or online.

Base Formula:

1   quart (4 cups) fresh or powdered goat's milk or unsweetened coconut milk (So Delicious™)
1   cup purified water
1-2 tsp nutritional or brewer's yeast
1-2 tsp unsulphured black strap molasses
¼   tsp kelp or trace minerals or 1/8 tsp sea salt
½   to ¾ capsule probiotic (Nature's Way Primadophilus Bifidus, keep refrigerated)
1-2 TBSP pure maple syrup

Additional Nutrients (Add 2-3 Times a Week):

1   TBSP total of any of these oils: cod liver oil, extra virgin olive oil, coconut oil, flax seed oil
¼   cup hemp protein powder (this can be taken every day for protein source)

Preparation:

Place all the ingredients except the probiotic into a medium sized sauce pan, turn the stove top onto medium low heat, place the pan on the stove, and stir until the ingredients are mixed. Do not over heat the formula; it should be slightly warm to the touch. Then after taking it off the stove, stir in the probiotic. Store the formula in a clean glass jar for up to 7-10 days. Two to three times a week add oil to the formula. One to two days a week add hemp protein (this step is not necessary unless your child is extremely deficient or you believe he/she would benefit from having extra protein).

Elderberry Cough and Immune Booster

Ingredients:

1 cup elderberry (dried), or 2 cups fresh
1 cinnamon stick
5 cloves
1 tablespoon of ginger root (freshly grated)

2 cups water preferably distilled but filtered is fine
1 cup raw honey, or maple syrup

Preparations:

Combine all ingredients except the raw honey into a small pot. Place on stovetop and bring to a boil on medium-high heat. Once it has started to boil, cover and reduce heat to simmer. Simmer for 20 to 30 minutes or until the liquid has been reduced by half.

Strain the simmered berry mixture into a bowl. Mash the berries with a spoon to extract more of the liquid. Add 1 cup of raw honey or maple syrup to the warm elderberry liquid. Wisk all together and pour into a clean mason jar with lid. You can use immediately or store in your refrigerator. Label the jar "Elderberry Immune Cough Syrup" and the date.

STORAGE: in a closed jar in the refrigerator for up to 2 months.

NOTE: Can be taken daily as a preventative measure and to fight off cold symptoms.

DOSAGE: Adults: 1 tablespoon daily as preventative, or 1 tablespoon every couple hours during cold symptoms. Children ages 4-10: take half the adult dosage and amount. Children under 4: take ¼ the adult dosage. Infants should not have honey until they are one years old.

Simple Elderberry Syrup – Immune Booster

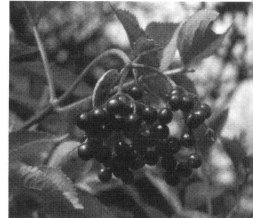

This is a great remedy for cold and flu prevention, (and at the onset), chest congestion and coughs. TIP: Let this sit overnight, at which time it will be ready in the morning!

Ingredients

1 cup dried elderberries
3.5 cups purified water.

Preparations:

Add about 1 full cup of dried elderberries to a quart mason jar. If you want to make a larger batch, adjust the quantity of berries so that the jar is 1/4 full. Add boiling water to the berries and completely fill the jar. Screw the lid on tightly and allow it to brew/steep for at least 8 hours! You can make it in the evening and it will be ready in the morning. Strain out the berries and pour the remaining contents back into the mason jar. You can add your favorite juice concentrate to the desired level of sweetness (as long as there are no added sugars) otherwise use raw honey or stevia to desired sweetness. You can even add some powdered Vitamin C for an extra kick. Use this up within a week to 10 days. Label the jar and date it.

DOSAGE: At onset of flu like symptoms or chest congestion take 1 cup every two hours. For children 4 to 10 years of age take half the dose and children under 4 take ¼ the adult dose. For prevention enjoy a ½ cup in the morning and evening, for children ages 4 to 10 take half the dosage and children 4 and younger take ¼ dosage.

BENEFITS OF KEFIR

In addition to beneficial bacteria and yeast, kefir contains minerals and essential amino acids that help the body with healing and maintenance functions. The complete proteins in kefir are already partially digested and therefore more easily utilized by the body. Tryptophan, one of the essential amino acids abundant in kefir, is well known for its relaxing effect on the nervous system. Because kefir also offers an abundance of calcium and magnesium, which are also important minerals for a healthy nervous system, kefir can have a particularly profound calming effect on the nerves.

Kefir's ample supply of phosphorus, the second most abundant mineral in our bodies, helps utilize carbohydrates, fats, and proteins for cell growth, maintenance and energy.

Kefir is rich in Vitamin B12, B1, and Vitamin K. It is an excellent source of biotin, a B Vitamin which aids the body's assimilation of other B Vitamins, such as folic acid, pantothenic acid, and B12. The numerous benefits of maintaining adequate B vitamin intake range from regulation of the kidneys, liver and nervous system to helping relieve skin disorders, boost energy and promote longevity. Easily digested, it cleanses the intestines, provides beneficial bacteria and yeast, vitamins and minerals, and complete proteins. Because kefir is such a balanced and nourishing food, it contributes to a healthy immune system and has been used to help patients suffering from AIDS, chronic fatigue syndrome, herpes, and cancer. Its tranquilizing effect on the nervous system has benefited many who suffer from sleep disorders, depression, and ADHD (attention deficit hyperactivity disorder).

The regular use of kefir can help relieve all intestinal disorders, promote bowel movement, reduce flatulence and create a healthier digestive system. In addition, its cleansing effect on the whole body helps to establish a balanced inner ecosystem for optimum health and longevity. Kefir can also help eliminate unhealthy food cravings by making the body more nourished and balanced. Its excellent nutritional content offers healing and health-maintenance benefits to people in every type of condition.

Coconut Milk Kefir

Great for upset stomach, bloating, indigestion and food allergies. Note: make sure to sterilize glass jars in boiling water before using.

Ingredients:

1 liter of coconut water
1 can of organic light coconut milk

1 packet of kefir starter.
Large gallon glass jar

Preparation:

Pour all 3 items into a large mouth gallon glass or plastic jar; It is not recommend to use metal because it will impede the bacteria's fermenting process. Pour the liquids into the jar and add the kefir grain starter. Stir gently with a plastic or wooden spoon. Place the lid on top and place into a basin of warm water at 90° F in order to raise the temperature of the mixture to 90°. Keep it warm in a dark cupboard, wrapped in some towels or a cooler to keep it at a steady temperature above 72° for 36 hours (for the first time starting the mixture). Never drink directly from the jar (pour the kefir into a separate cup) and do not place a dirty spoon into the jar, otherwise you greatly reduce the quality and quantity of the probiotics in the kefir.

After 36 hours, the kefir has activated. Give it a stir with a clean plastic spatula and it will be ready to drink. Start by drinking 1-2 oz. and increase to 4 oz daily. Place the kefir into the fridge, and use up within 5-7 days.

For future batches up to six times (if using a packet starter) allow it to sit for 24 hours. To start a new batch of kefir, take 6 TBSP of the bottom matter of the original batch and place into the next batch.

Coconut Water Kefir

Great for upset stomach, bloating, indigestion and food allergies. Note: make sure to sterilize glass jars in boiling water before using.

Ingredients:

1 liter of coconut water
1 packet of kefir starter
Liter Glass Mason Jar

Preparation:

Pour the liquids into the jar and add the kefir grain starter. Stir gently with a plastic or wooden spoon. Place the lid on top and place into a basin of warm water at 90° F in order to raise the temperature of the mixture to 90°. Then keep it warm in a dark cupboard, wrapped in some towels or a cooler to keep it at a steady temperature above 72° for 36 hours, for the first time starting the mixture. Never drink directly from the jar (pour the kefir into a separate cup) and do not place a dirty spoon into the jar, otherwise you greatly reduce the quality and quantity of the probiotics in the kefir.

After the kefir has activated, give it a stir with a clean plastic spatula and it is ready to be consumed. Start of by drinking 1-2 oz. and increase to 4 oz daily. Place the kefir into the fridge, and use up within 5-7 days.

For future batches up to six times (if using a packet starter) you will allow the mix to activate for 24 hours. To restart a new batch of kefir, take 6 TBSP of the bottom matter of the original batch and place into the next batch.

Your Eating Style--Shopping Guide

Ironically, the cost of eating organic foods has become exorbitant. A more practical solution and one that will make shopping for organic foods exciting and light on your budget is a food makeover. Use this chapter to guide your makeover and help you in make wholesome choices. If you follow this plan you can cut your costs dramatically. Here are some questions to answer before you begin:

- What is the desired food budget?
- What locally grown produce can be found in your neighborhood?
- Is there a food share program or coop offered by local farmers?
- If there is no local food market cooperative available, turn to the local health food store.

First, we want to plan our weekly menu--planning ahead will help us cut costs and improve our health. By having a plan, we are less likely to purchase packaged snack foods. Before we make our list we should ask ourselves these questions: What foods do we really need? What is my personal snack habit costing me in dollars and in health? Can I trade garden produce with another neighbor? Will picking up a calendar or printing out a free calendar online help me to lay out a week or month food plan?

First, try to buy items in bulk whole quantities. Second, buy locally produced items first. Third, make sure we have the necessary tools to use on the items that are purchased. Other suggestions: stock up when items are on sale, then freeze, blanch and freeze, or can foods for the winter months.

The cost of eating organically becomes more manageable when we replace our snack foods, low in nutritional value, with healthier choices. There are comparisons listed below so that you can see the differences.

THE COST OF SMART SHOPPING, MAKES YOU HEALTHIER

Check out these simple comparisons:

1. One 8 oz. bag of organic potato chips can cost anywhere from $3.50-4.99; whereas a 1 lb. bag of organic red potatoes costs around a $1.79.

2. One 4 oz. bag of rice crackers is $3.50 whereas a 1 lb. bag of organic brown rice costs between $1.25-2.00.

3. Breakfast price for a family of four over the course of a year:

- One 50 lb. bag of organic steel cut oats retails for about $64.99, which can feed a family of four at 1/2 cup dried (which is 300 calories) per person for 65 days. This initial investment of $64.99 costs only $1 dollar a day, **or $365.00 a year**.
  OR
- Quaker Apples & Cinnamon Instant Oatmeal, each serving of which is 130 calories. To reach the 300 calorie baseline, each person will need 2 1/2 packs, which equals 1 case a morning for a family of four (if there are 10 packs in a case). This costs $4.29 per meal, and for 2 months it costs $267.15. Over the course of a year, breakfast would cost your family **$1,565.85**.
- In one year of buying steel cut oats, we save **$1,200**. Not only have we made healthier choices but we have saved our family an outstanding amount of money.

When making the decision to replace food(s), really think carefully what is best for you and your family. For example, if you must choose between switching to organic cereal or organic mayonnaise, and your kids go through two boxes of cereal a week, but only four tablespoons of mayo a week, change the cereal. The cheaper, healthier source would be to buy oatmeal in bulk or make your own granola. Improve your health and keep your costs down through growing, buying, and eating unrefined, organic foods in their original state, the way God intended. Shopping organically does not need to be expensive; if you have the option, buy in bulk, buy foods in season, join a food club, or start your own garden.

KNOW YOUR LABELS

In today's market there is little accountability for the labeling of our foods. This mislabeling manipulates buyers into thinking they are getting more for their money, a healthier product or whole foods. In North America, Genetically Modified Foods (GMO's) are not required to carry a label that says GMO. Currently, the only way a consumer can avoid GMO foods with certainty is to buy only organic. Hopefully the organic label will never be degraded to the point where we cannot rely on it to avoid GMO. Soy, canola, cotton (cottonseed), and corn (including popcorn), are all genetically modified, unless the product or food says " certified organic" or "non-GMO". This means that any product you purchase with any of these ingredients contains GMO's, including soy products, corn syrup, low-fat frozen dinners, and canola and soy oil which are frequently in baked goods, salad dressings, and mixed spices. We recommend that you select only foods classified as organic, biodynamic, or grown from heirloom seeds if possible.

Monosodium Glutamate (MSG) has many names and combinations. Listed on the following page are the names of ingredients that contain enough MSG to trigger an allergic or negative health reaction. Be on the lookout for deceptive food packaging!

HIDDEN NAMES OF MSG:

ALWAYS contain a form of MSG:	Often Contain MSG or create MSG during processing:
Natural flavor(s)	Carrageenan
Natural flavoring(s)	Maltodextrin
Natural colors	Malt extract
Glutamate	Natural pork flavoring
Glutamic acid	Citric acid
Gelatin	Malt flavoring
Monosodium glutamate	Bouillon
Calcium caseinate	Broth natural
Textured protein	Chicken flavoring
Monopotassium glutamate	Soy protein isolate
Sodium caseinate	Natural beef flavoring
Yeast nutrient	Non-fat dry milk
Yeast extract	Ultra-pasteurized
Yeast food	Soy sauce stock
Autolyzed yeast	Barley malt
Hydrolyzed protein (any protein that is hydrolyzed)	Soy sauce extract
Hydrolyzed corn gluten	Whey protein concentrate
Natrium glutamate (natrium is Latin/German for sodium)	Soy protein
	Whey protein
	Protease
	Soy protein concentrate
	Whey protein isolate
	Protease enzymes
	Anything protein fortified
	Flavors(s) & flavoring(s)
	Anything enzyme modified

Learn more about food labeling at: www.truthinlabeling.org/index.html and www.msgtruth.org/whatisit.htm

UNFIT FOODS TO AVOID

Always read the label! If the product contains anything listed below, it is not healthy for you, and is robbing your body of life and health. The more of these ingredients included the more harm it does to your body. Don't just look at calorie amounts from fat, sugar, carbohydrates, and protein as they only tell you part of the story. You need to look at the full story and read the ingredients! Use wisdom when shopping as flashy products can make claims like "fat-free, low-sodium, sugar-free, high-protein, all natural," but are far from being healthy for you. Take your time while shopping; be smart when choosing products and you will start to see the difference.

Oils and Fats

Hydrogenated Oil
Rapeseed Oil
Margarine
Vegetable Oil
Animal Lard
Soy Butter

Corn Oil
Peanut Oil
Partially-Hydrogenated Oil
Canola Oil
Non-organic Butter

Preservatives

Salt & Refined Sea Salt
Sulfur Dioxide
Distilled Vinegar
Chloride
Artificial Flavors
White Vinegar
BHT
Natural Flavors

Potassium Sorbate
Artificial Colors
MSG
Hydrolyzed Yeast
Ferrous Fumerate
Spices
EDTA

Sugars

Corn Syrup
Refined Honey
Sweet & Low
White Sugar
Fructose
Aspartame

Brown Sugar
Glucose
Sucralose
High Fructose Corn Syrup
Refined Cane Sugar
Corn Syrup

Miscellaneous Foods

The items marked with an * are okay to use if they are organic. Organic goat milk derived products are healthy in moderation.

Highly Refined Foods
Graham Crackers
Buttermilk*
Soy Protein Isolate
Packaged Frosting
Sour Cream
Bleached Wheat Flour
Sugar Cereals
Cornmeal*
Unbleached Wheat Flour
Puddings
Enriched Flour

Catsup/Ketchup
Corn*
Enriched Products
Milk Peanuts
Mayonnaise
Butter
Wheat Gluten
Pasteurized Cheese
Processed Meats, Deli Meat
Vital Wheat Gluten
Peanut Butter

Beverages

The items below that are marked with an * are acceptable when organic; however, it is not necessarily a food to use frequently or a food to give you restored health. Organic coffee is a healthier alternative to non-organic; however, it should not be used on a daily basis.

Decaf Coffee
Carbonated Beverages
Hard Liquor
Tap Water
Energy Drinks
Soy Milk

Wines with Added Sugar
Fruit Juices (with sugar)*
Black Tea
Soda/Pop
Pasteurized Milk
Non-Organic Coffee

WHAT LABELS MEAN (According to the USDA):

100 percent organic:
Products that are completely organic or made of all organic ingredients. Buying organic is the safest and best choice when buying foods.

Organic:
Products that are at least 95 percent organic.

Made with organic ingredients:
These are products that contain at least 70 percent organic ingredients. The organic seal can't be used on these packages.

Free Range:
The USDA defines this to mean birds (poultry) are allowed access to the outdoors for more than half their lives. However, just because the cage door was open doesn't mean the birds actually spent time outside. This claim is not independently verified.

Grass Fed:
According to the USDA, the label means the animal consumed only grass or forage throughout its adult life, was fed no grain, and had continuous access to pasture during the growing season.

Natural:
According to the USDA, food can only be labeled natural if it contains no artificial ingredients or added colors and is minimally processed. For meat and poultry, the "natural" label applies to how meat is processed, not how animals are raised. For example, animal products raised with the use of artificial hormones can be labeled natural. So can genetically modified organisms.

Food Product Code:
The following are some food labeling items you will want to consider when shopping for groceries. These are usually on a sticker that is found on fruits and vegetables. Look at the product sticker to determine what quality of food the product may be.

If the first number of five is a 9, the produce is organic.
If the first number of five is an 8, it is GMO or from a genetically modified source.
If there are only four numbers, the produce is conventional, meaning not organic.

The following foods marked with a + are **heavily sprayed with pesticides** if purchased conventionally (meaning non-organic). Health food stores like Wild Oats, Whole Foods, Vitamin Cottage, and Sunflower Market carry a variety of these foods, however, organic foods are becoming more readily available in your local grocery store (although they are sometimes a bit pricier). Vitamin

Cottage or your local health food store will most likely have more reasonable prices than the larger chain health food stores. You will want to check out several stores and compare their selection, quality, and price with one another; make sure to be careful of markets that mix organic with conventional! In the lists that follow, parentheses indicate the best brands found thus far; however, this is not an exhaustive list. Check out **www.living-foods.com/articles/twelvelist.html** for more helpful info.

FOOD BEAUTIFUL SHOPPING LIST

GRAINS, FLOURS & BREADS

While you are out shopping keep in mind to buy organic grains in bulk, which are higher in nutritional value and have no pesticides and herbicides on them. When you get home, make sure to store these grains in your refrigerator or freezer so they do not spoil. For advice on long term storage you can check out this website: **http://beprepared.com**. Some grains you should avoid are non-organic wheat, corn, and their flour forms. Non-organic wheat flour spoils within two weeks of milling, making it very toxic for you. Sprouted grain is the best form of bread to eat as it has three times more nutritional value than flour breads and is much easier to digest. Alvarado St. Bakery and Food for Life are some companies that make excellent sprouted grain breads, bagels, tortillas, and pasta.

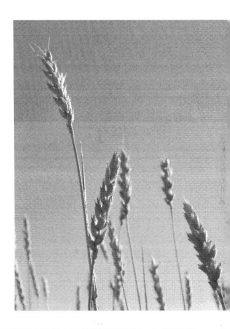

Sample Shopping List

- Amaranth
- Oat Groats
- Rolled Oats
- Steel Cut Oats
- Quinoa
- Spelt Flour
- Spelt Grain
- Kamut (Rolled)
- Tritical Flakes
- Sprouted Grain Bread

- Brown Rice
- Brown Rice Flour
- Sweet Brown Rice
- Rye Grain
- Rye Flour
- Coconut Flour
- Almond Flour
- Teff
- Buckwheat
- Tapioca Flour/Grain

FRUITS & FRUIT JUICES

Some of the fruits below can also be purchased frozen by Stahlbush or Cascadian Farms. For fruit juices, always dilute with purified water (1 to 3, water to juice), and choose from brands such as Knudson, Santa Cruz, or Lakewood Organics.

Sample Shopping List

- Apples
- Apricots +
- Bananas
- Kiwi fruit
- Figs
- Prunes
- Dates
- Raisins +
- Limes
- Nectarines
- Melons
- Mangoes
- Pineapples
- Papayas

- Grapefruits
- Lemons
- Avocados +
- Grapes (Seeded)
- Strawberries +
- Blueberries
- Pears
- Peaches +
- Blackberries
- Raspberries
- Cranberries
- Tangerines
- Tomatoes +

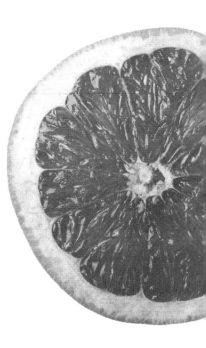

VEGETABLES

I highly encourage you to purchase all foods organic because many of the conventional vegetables are genetically modified. Those marked with a + are *definitely genetically modified* unless they are organic.

Sample Shopping List

- Alfalfa Sprouts
- Artichoke
- Asparagus
- Baby Corn +
- Bamboo Shoots
- Beets
- Beet Greens

- Bell Peppers
- Broccoli +
- Cabbage
- Carrots
- Cauliflower
- Celery
- Chicory

- Chili Pepper
- Chives
- Collard Greens
- Cucumber +
- Dandelion Greens
- Eggplant
- Endive
- Escarole
- Garlic
- Ginger
- Horseradish
- Jicama
- Kale
- Lettuce
- Leeks
- Mushrooms (Portabello, Shitakii)
- Mustard Greens
- Onion
- Okra

- Parsley
- Parsnips
- Potatoes (Red) +
- Pumpkin
- Radish
- Rutabaga
- Shallots
- Sorrel
- Spinach
- Sprouts
- Squash
- Sugar Snap Peas
- Swiss Chard
- Taro Root
- Turnip
- Water chestnuts
- Watercress
- Yellow Squash
- Zucchini

UNPASTUERIZED DAIRY & NON-DAIRY

Try to avoid items that are enriched with vitamins, as these products contain synthetic vitamins which deplete your body of nutrients. Also, try and keep canola-based oil products to a minimum and use the healthier recommended oils listed under Fantastic Food Replacements.

Sample Shopping List

- Coconut Milk (So Delicious™)
- Coconut Kefir and Yogurt
- Rice Milk (Vanilla or Plain)
- Hemp Milk
- Oat Milk (Pacific™)
- Multi Grain Milk (Pacific™)
- Almond Milk

- Organic Goat Yogurt
- Chocolate Chips (Tropical Source™, Sunspire™)
- Carob Chips (Sunspire™)
- Rice, Almond, Vegan cheese
- Raw Goat Cheese (Organic Valley™)

HEALTHY OILS

Choose cold-pressed organic oils because they are not heated up to extract the oil. This preserves the nutrients and healing properties of the oil. Oils should be used minimally at all times, and the best way to eat healthy oils is in its original food state. For example, use ground flax seed instead of consuming the oil.

- Virgin Coconut Oil (Jungle Life™)
- Extra Virgin Olive Oil (Olio Beato,
        Omega Nutrition)
- Flax Seed Oil (Barlean's Organics)

- Hempseed Oil (Manitoba Harvest)
- Sesame Oil (Flora, Spectrum)
- Sunflower & Walnut Oil (Spectrum)
- Organic Butter (Organic Valley)

The best oil for cooking is coconut oil!

Oil substitutes for sautéing: apple sauce, sherry, vegetable stock, vinegars, wine, beer, low-sodium Tamari (soy-sauce).

Oil substitutes for baking: applesauce, pureed bananas, pureed stewed prunes.
Use citrus juices in place of salad dressing, or apple cider vinegar, tomato sauce, or no-oil dressings.

PROTEIN SOURCES

Many of the foods in other categories (seeds, nuts, vegetables, grains, etc.) have amino acids, which make up protein structures in the body. Food Beautiful is a plant-based eating style that promotes using plants for the primary nutrient source. Sometimes animal-based foods can be medicinal for you; however, this does not mean you need meat as your medicine. Animal foods are meant for individuals with extremely low body weight and malnourishment. Most people are not dealing with this kind of condition. Always avoid eating any meat while dining out, since you have little control on source and quality. If you are addicted to meat or dairy, try cutting the amount you normally eat in half, and then limit it to one time a week, with your end goal being once or twice a month.

- Sprouted grains, seeds, lentils, alfalfa, broccoli, radish
- Avocados
- Seeds (hemp, sunflower, sesame, pumpkin, chia)
- Nuts (almonds, cashews, brazil, walnuts, pecans)
- Quinoa and buckwheat
- Raw goat milk
- Tempe (fermented soy beans)
- Eggs (organic/free range/roaming)
- Freshwater or wild caught fish (salmon, halibut, yellow perch, trout, tuna, herring,
        bass, cod, haddock)

- Free range buffalo (www.wildideabuffalo.com or www.eatbisonmeat.com)
- Venison & elk meat
- Organic lamb (www.organiclamb.com, www.rockyplains.com, or www.foxfirefarms.com)

NUTS & SEEDS

Buy raw organic as much as possible. Keep all your de-shelled nuts and seeds refrigerated as they can go rancid (spoil) quickly if unshelled. I do not recommend roasted nuts or seeds (with exception to pumpkin seeds) as this causes them to lose their vitamin E (which protects the other vitamins and minerals in the nut/seed) and denatures the quality of the natural oils within them.

Sample Shopping List

- Almonds (Raw)
- Coconut Meal
- Coconut Flakes (Without Sugar)
- Chia Seeds (Raw)
- Brazil Nuts (Raw)
- Cashews (Raw)
- Chestnuts (Seasonal, Boiled)
- Pecans (Raw)

- Hazelnuts (Raw)
- Walnuts (Raw)
- Pumpkin Seeds (Roasted or Raw)
- Black Sesame Seeds (Raw)
- Sesame Seeds (Raw & Unhulled)
- Sunflower Seeds (Raw)
- Poppy Seeds (Raw)
- Flax Seed (Raw or Ground)

BEANS & LEGUMES

Beans can be found in whole form, bulk, flours, and in cans. You can sprout beans to increase their mineral, amino-acid, and enzymatic composition by soaking them in water overnight. The next morning discard the excess water and rinse the beans.

Sample Shopping List

- Aduki & Sprouts
- Adzuki
- Black Beans
- Bean Sprouts
- Organic Refried Beans
- Green Lentils
- Red Lentils

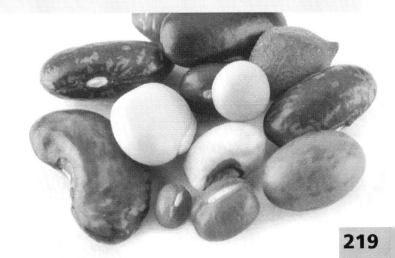

- Yellow Lentils
- Garbanzo Beans/Chickpeas
- Kidney Beans
- Black Eyed Peas & Sprouts

- Navy Beans
- Lima Beans
- Mung Beans & Sprouts
- Peas

PACKAGED FOODS

- Brown Rice Noodles (Thai Kitchen, Tinkyada)
- Kamut Noodles (Cleopatra's Noodles, Eden Organics)
- Spelt Pasta & Noodles (by VitaSpelt)
- Sprouted Noodles and Pastas (Food For Life)
- Bean Noodles
- Rice Cakes (by Lunberg)
- Rice Crackers (Hol-Grain, Edward & Sons, San-J)
- Blue & Red Corn Chips (by Kettle, Guiltless Gourmet)
- Potato Chips made with Oive Oil (Kettle, Terra-Red Bliss)
- Cheeto Replacement (Tings by Robert's American Gourmet)
- Cookies (Enjoy Life, Small Planet Foods)
- Flax Crackers (Foods Alive--order at Foodbeautiful.com)
- Amaranth Crackers (Nu World Foods)
- Healthy Bars (Organic Food Bar, Lara Bars, BubbleBar's)
- Chocolate Bars (Dagoba, Endangered Species, Newman's Organics)

CONDIMENTS

It seems as though more products are adding canola oil, which is a hybrid seed oil that has high amounts of Omega 6's, which, in excess, can cause physical problems. It is not recommended that you use canola oil regularly; it can cause cholesterol and plaque to build up in your arteries, and cause arthritic-type symptoms. Here are some healthier alternatives:

- Ranch Dressing (Tammy's Second Chance Ranch)
- Applesauce from organic apples (Solana Gold, Santa Cruz)
- Mustard made with Apple Cider Vinegar (Annie's Natural)
- Apple Cider Vinegar (Bragg)
- Liquid Aminos (Bragg)
- Almond Butter (Raw) (Maranatha)

- Tahini (Raw) (Maranatha)
- Brewer's Yeast (Lewis Labs, KAL)
- Lemon Juice (Lakewood Organic, Santa Cruz)
- Jams (Fruit Sweetened) (St. Daflour, Crofters, Fiordifrutta)
- Honey (Raw) (Ambrosia, Really Raw Honey, Clark's Raw Honey)
- Maple Syrup (Shady Maple)
- Sucanat (Unrefined Sugar)
- Date Sugar
- Coconut Sugar
- Black Strap Molasses (Unsulphured) (by Plantations)
- Stevia (Liquid or Powder) (Now, Sweet Leaf)
- Rice Sour Cream (Rice)
- Mayonnaise Replacement (Vegannaise by Follow your Heart™)
- Salsa (505 Organics, Emerald Valley Kitchen)
- Ketchup (Fruit Juice Sweetened) (by Muir Glen Organics)
- Green Chili (Pork Free) (505 Organics)
- Red Chile Sauce (505 Organics)
- Coconut Milk (Nature's Forest)
- Xylitol (Ultimate Sweetener™ , Emerald Forest™ , KAL™)

TEA

Making tea is easier than you may think. Use fresh picked herbs for teas and/or buy organic store-bought blends. Get creative with your teas! If you have a garden, use the leaves or flowers from the plants. You can even make tea from the bulk herbs and spices that are available at health food stores. Sip on your garden herbs (dandelion-all parts, rosemary leaves, basil leaves, lavender flower, echinacea flower, raspberry leaves, baby rose buds, mint) by themselves or alongside green tea. Thyme and oregano tea is especially good for colds and killing germs, plus it is very soothing and tastes great with a little honey. With extra fruits around you can add a few blueberries, a bit of strawberry, or some citrus rind. Get creative with using left-over fruit and fruit rinds in your tea.

Boiling water is simple and fast. Simply pour boiling water over herbs and let steep between 3-7 minutes depending on how strong you like your tea. The longer the herb sits in the water the more bitter it can become. After boiling the water and steeping, use a colander to drain out the herbs before drinking. Here is where a French press comes in handy or otherwise just use a colander. You may want to sweeten your tea with xylitol or raw honey.

Mix and match the herbs below, or others you may have in your garden or pantry.

Herbs & Fruits For Tea:	Herbal Teas:	Good Brands:
Citrus Rinds	Milk Thistle	Yogi Teas
Berry Fruits	Dandelion	Alvita Teas
Lemon Thyme	Ginger	Celestial Seasoning (Organic Line)
Lemon Grass	Red Raspberry Leaves	St. Daflour
Parsley & Lemon	Mint Leaves	Lotus Island
Cranberry	Oregano	Traditional Medicinal
Rose Bud Blossoms	Basil	
Chamomile	Echinacea Flower	
Cinnamon	Peppermint	

SPICES & HERBS

If you have had your spices for more than a year, replace them with fresh herbs. You can store spices in the freezer to preserve their effectiveness, freshness, and taste, otherwise, use your cupboard spices within a year from purchasing. Simply Organic, Frontier, Spice Island and The Spice Hunter are the best brand names to purchase from. Feel free to purchase spices that are premixed for Mexican, Thai, and Italian dishes. Make sure that none of your spices has ingredients such as salt, MSG, spices, or "natural flavors" in them as these are neurotoxins that stimulate your hypothalamus (taste center of your brain) to crave more food. Always remember that any vegetable meal can transform from boring to fabulous by adding more spices, stevia, or fruit juice.

Sample Shopping List

- Anise	- Cloves	- Peppermint
- Dill	- Cinnamon	- Paprika
- Sage	- Cayenne Pepper	- Lemon Balm
- Ginger	- Chili Pepper	- Marjoram
- Fennel	- Lemon Peel	- Orange Oil
- Cumin	- White Pepper	- Tarragon
- Celery Seed	- Licorice	- Turmeric
- Coriander	- Spearmint	- Sea Salt (Redmond's)
- Cardamom		

NUTRITIONAL SUPPLEMENTS

This is a list of the supplements I recommend and use myself, as they are the highest quality around, free of toxins and pollutants. You can some of these products on my website (**www.FoodBeautiful.com**). Other products can be ordered by calling the company directly or plugging their name into your internet search engine. You can order the AIM products by calling 1-800-456-2462 and giving them referral #591683. This will give you the products at cost. Many of these supplements are ones we suggest to our clients. There are also products available on our websites that are not on the list below.

- Zrii (Zrii)

- Sea Minerals - Supaboost, Stinging Nettles, Hawthorn (www.foodbeautiful.com)

- Ultimate Superfood - Pure Synergy (The Synergy Company)

- Klamath Crystals (The Synergy Company)

- Turmeric Force (New Chapter)

- EFA's - Omega 3's (Nutri-West, Carlson's)

- Cod Liver Oil – Omega 3's and Vitamin D (Carlson's)

- Multivitamin - Food Based (The Synergy Company, Innate – www.foodbeautiful.com)

- Probiotic (AIM, New Chapter, Threelac)

- Digestive Enzymes (AIM, ReNew Life Formulas)

- Amino Acids (Nutri-West, Green Herb)

- Calcium from Living Food Source (Innate, VegLife, Brazil Coral Calcium, Green Herb)

- Liquid Iron - Food Derived Source (Floridix)

- Barley Greens Powder - Barley Life (AIM)

- Leafy Greens Powder (AIM)

- Carrot Powder (AIM)

- Anti-Parasitical, Colon Cleaner - Herbal Fiber Blend (AIM)

- Anti Viral, Bacterial - Oil of Oregano & Olive Leaf Extract (GAIA)

- Miracle Mineral Solution, MMS (www.foodbeautiful.com)

RESOURCE GUIDE FOR PURCHASES:

Raw and Organic Foods & Herbs:

www.realrawfood.com

www.herbwisdom.com

Highest-quality raw, fermented, and cultured vegetables:

REJUVENATE FOODS
800-805-7957
www.rejuvinate.com

Packaged and bulk organic grains and flours:

ARROWHEAD MILLS
(800) 749-0730
www.arrowheadmills.com

Raw foods, snacks, live food supplements, juicers, blenders, and many other excellent products:

THE RAW WORLD
P.O. Box 16156
West Palm Beach, FL 33416
866-RAW DIET
www.therawworld.com

Organic raw nuts, seeds, and butters:

GLASER ORGANICS
19100 SW 137th Ave
Miami, FL 33012
305-238-7747
www.glaserorganicfarm.com

Raw organic goat dairy products; raw cheeses, milk and yogurt; free range turkey, goat, and beef:

WHITE EGRET FARM
512-267-7408
www.whiteegretfarm.com

Organic Wine Resources:

Certified organic, biodynamic, and sulfite-free wines:

PLEASANT VALLEY WINERY
541-387-3040
www.pheasantvalleywinery.com

ECO VINE CLUB
805-688-4455
www.ecovinewine.com

WILBUR'S TOTAL BEVARAGE
Fort Collins, CO
888-988-WINE
www.wilburstotalbeverage.com

COPPER MOUNTAIN WINES
503-649-0027
www.coopermountainwine.com

FRE VINEYARDS
800-760-3739
www.frewine.com

How to Store Foods:

www.gardenguides.com/how-to/tipstechniques/
vegetables/storing.asp
www.frugalsquirrels.com

How to Find Local Farms:

www.localharvest.org

Nut, Herb, Grain Grinders:

www.countrylivinggrainmills.com

Free Range Meat and Wild Salmon:

Certified organic, free-range poultry:

COLLEGE HILL POULTRY
220 North Center St.
Fredericksburg, PA 17026
www.raisedright.com

Organic grass-feed beef and wild salmon; raw dairy products: butter, yogurt, kefir and cheese:

REAL FOODS MARKET
743 West 1200 North, Suite 200
Springville, UT 84663
886-284-7325
www.realfoodsmarket.com

Wild sockeye salmon:

BRISTOL BAY
207-223-4353
www.bristolbaywildsalmon.com

Organic foods of all varieties:

EAT WILD
www.eatwild.com

ORGANIC VALLEY
507 W. Main St.
LaFarge, WI 54639
608-625-2602
www.organicvalley.com

Grow Your Own Garden:

gardening.about.com

www.organicgardening.com/

www.sacgardens.org/

journeytoforever.org/garden.html

www.sacgardens.org/sustaingarden.html

Research what produce you can grow in your climate and geographical region. Factors which will determine what and how much you can grow include: soil conditions, the amount of sunlight, and the amount of property you are capable of devoting to a vegetable garden.

Food Replacements

Unfit foods, foods which are highly processed, cooked, altered, acidic, or containing a high glycemic index, should be omitted from your diet. The left column below contains a list of foods you should avoid, foods that can cause allergies and toxicity while encouraging diseases to permeate the body. The foods on the right are healthy sources that encourage a healthy eating style. Most people with candida and cancer should eliminate animal-based foods and sugars, with the exception of xylitol and stevia from their diet. Those with diabetes should avoid foods with high glycemic sugars, like honey and raw cane sugar. This is not an exhaustive list of foods to eliminate from your diet, but a strong guide that will help you begin to build your beautiful eating style.

AVOID This Unfit Food	USE this Instead
High Fructose Corn Syrup	Unsulfured Black Strap Molasses
Corn Syrup	Brown Rice Syrup
Brown Sugar	Sucanat (unrefined raw cane sugar)
White Sugar	Xylitol (non-GMO) Stevia Powder Sucanat (unrefined raw cane sugar)
Refined Honey	Raw Unfiltered Honey Local Raw Honey
Aspartame, Sucralose	Organic Stevia Powder Organic Stevia Liquid
Milk	Unsweetened Coconut Milk Unsweetened Almond Milk Hemp Milk
Cheese	Raw Goat Cheese Almond, Rice Cheese Vegan Cheese
Yogurt	Coconut Kefir and Yogurt Goat Yogurt and Kefir
Sour Cream	Goat Yogurt Rice Sour Cream (by Rice™)
Butter	Virgin Red Palm Oil Virgin Coconut Oil
Meat	Veggie Burgers Tempe Soft Boil Eggs Nuts and Seeds
Mayonnaise	Vegannaise™, Nayonnaise™
Ketchup	Fruit Sweetened Ketchup
Natural Flavors	Organic "Plant Derived" Flavor
Natural Colors	Organic "Plant Derived" Colors
Spices	Organic Spices
MSG	Sea Salt and Plant Derived Spices From Your Pantry

GRAINS

There are a number of highly nutrient-dense grains available that can be used instead of wheat. Non-organic wheat can harbor myotoxins and bacteria, and processing the grains without refrigeration causes it to go rancid within two weeks of milling. This process is toxic for the body. If you do use wheat choose the organic wheat. If you are gluten intolerant or allergic to wheat you can use any of the "Best Replacements" except for spelt and barley. All other grains are low in gluten, which means they will not raise the same in the baking process, so next to each replacement is their suggested use.

When selecting grains to purchase, buy them in bulk, because this will save you money and increase the nourishment of your meals. You will want to buy 25 lb. bags, place 2-5 lbs. in a large jar in your kitchen, then store the remaining portion in sealed Mylar bags inside large plastic buckets.

The following page lists quality organic replacements for wheat, corn and low-nutrient grains, along with their uses.

For information on how to store grains, visit **www.frugalsquirrels.com**. Learn about grain grinders at **www.countrylivinggrainmills.com**. I recommend buying a stainless steel grain grinder that is guaranteed to last a lifetime. I prefer the Country Living Mill that does not run on electricity, has different grinding sizes, grinds almost anything, and is guaranteed to last longer than your lifetime.

TIPS

Foods that act as binders:
Eggs, mashed potato, arrowroot, psyllium seed husk powder, ground flax seed, pectin, whole chia seed, silken tofu, tapioca flour, and banana.

Gluten-free grains:
Brown rice flour, sweet brown rice, buckwheat, quinoa, non-gluten sources of oats, sorghum, tapioca, teff, kamut, rye, millet, arrowroot, and xantham gum.

Oil replacements in baking:
Applesauce, goat yogurt, coconut milk, and discarded juicer pulp.

AVOID	BEST REPLACEMENT	SUGGESTED USES
Wheat	Amaranth Grain/Flour	Crackers, pie crusts, waffles, quick breads
	Rolled Oats & Flour	Zucchini bread, cake, muffins, crackers, cookies
	Kamut Flour	Pizza crust, bread, muffins, cookies
	Buckwheat Flour	Pancakes, thickener
	Quinoa Grain/Flour	Muffins, cookies, pancakes, pilaf
	Rye Grain/Flour	Bread, crusts, pancakes, waffles, cookies
	Garbanzo Bean Flour	Muffins, pancakes, quick breads
	Fava Bean Flour	Flat bread, pancakes
	Tapioca Flour/Grain	Binder, pudding, pancakes, sugar cookies
Wheat, Cornmeal	Brown Rice/Flour	Scones, bread; needs binder
Wheat Flour	Teff	Flat bread, muffins, pie crust; needs binder
	Barley Flour	Breads, muffins, cakes
	Spelt Flour	Pie crust, bread, cookies, puff pie
Wheat Grains	Spelt Grain	Grain cereals, pilaf, hot cereal
Wheat Grits	Oat Groats or Steel Cut Rolled Oats & Flour	Cookies, cereal, crackers
Corn, Cornmeal	Millet	Corn meal, corn bread, flat bread
Wheat & White Rice	Buclwheat	Pilaf, side dish
White Rice	Sweet Brown Rice	Muffins, side dishes, salads,
Nut Flours	Coconut Flour/Flakes	Macaroons, cookies, cakes, salads
	Almond Flour	Cakes, pancakes, thickener
All Breads	Sprouted Bread	Sandwiches, croutons, toast
Thickeners	Xantham Gum	Thickener
Corn Starch	Arrowroot Flour	Thickener
Ground Cornmeal	Sorghum	Thickener

First Aid Food Kit--Foods That "Kill The Craving"

Need a fix for that sweet or salty tooth? You can minimize those unwanted cravings with foods that nurture the body. Sometimes you may need an easy chart to convert those bad meals into healthy meals for ideas. It's good to have the knowledge inside this book, but when your blood sugar is low and you are "jonesin" for a fix; this will be your first aid food kit.

The fun chart below lists ideal replacement foods across from their unhealthy low-nutrient counterpart. On the right are listed choice foods which have the vitamins and minerals your body is truly craving in order to satisfy that urge. If you know you have a specific craving, start making the recipes and you will see a noticeable reduction in the amount of binge eating or out-of-control

WHEN YOU CRAVE THIS	CHOOSE THIS
Homemade Apple Pie	Charosset * Raw Berry Pie * Sarah's Best Banana Bread Ever * Diced apples, dates, and chopped cashews
Brownies	Fudge Black Bean Brownies * Date Coconut Log *
Burritos	Veggie Tortilla Wrap * Low Carb Rolls * using 505 green chili sauce
Candy Bar	Chocolate Cashew Butter Cups * *Low cal option:* Lara Bar or Panda Licorice Date Coconut Logs *
Chips	RC-GC Salad * Kale Chips * Almond Crackers
Chip or Veggie Dip	Fire Roasted Hummus * Creamy Ranchero * Black beans puréed with salsa and seasonings

WHEN YOU CRAVE THIS	CHOOSE THIS
Chocolate or Fudge	Frozen banana, vegan dark chocolate Fruits For Immune Power Juice * Fudge Drops *
Cheese or Cheese Dip	Raw goat cheese Rice or almond cheese No Cheese Cheesy Dippin' Sauce *
Cookies	Chia Energy Cookies * Sarah's Best Banana Bread Ever * Lara Bar
Ranch Dressing or Dip	Veggie Ranch Dip *
Toast	Ezekiel bread toast with coconut oil Brown rice with sea salt and oil
Drugs, Alcohol, Cigarettes	Green Machine Juice * Bananas Chia tea Color Me A Rainbow Juice *
Relief from a Hangover	Real V-8 Juice * Body Cooler Juice * Tummy Tonic Juice * Carrot Lemon Juice * Clean As a Whistle Juice * 1 TBSP apple cider vinegar, 8 oz. water, 1 TBSP honey
Ice Cream	Mango Cream * Berry Blue Smoothie * Toasted Coconut Ice Cream *
Hamburger	Lentil Loaf with Barbecue Sauce * Simplest Veggie Burgers *
Mashed Potatoes and Gravy	Mashed Potato Makeover *

WHEN YOU CRAVE THIS	CHOOSE THIS
Hot Chocolate or Chocolate Milk	Coconut milk with cocoa powder, stevia or xylitol
French Fries	Sweet Potato Fries Roasted Baby Vegetables✳
Fried Foods	Foods Should Taste Good™ Chips Sunny side-up eggs on Ezekiel bread Sauteed vegetables (potatoes, yams, onion) in coconut oil, garlic, sea salt
Waffles	"BananaOat" Waffles✳ Mom's Puffed Pie✳
Pancakes	Oatmeal/kamut/spelt pancakes Mom's Puffed Pie✳
Pastries & Muffins	Multi-Grain Cereal✳ Walnut Raisin Breakfast Cake✳ Raw Oatmeal✳ Poppy Seed Muffins✳
Pizza	California Pizza Spelt Crust✳
Pop	Kombucha – guava, mango or berry flavor Knudson Juice™ with some club soda Freshly juiced fruit Zevia™ Ginger Ale✳
Pudding	Dairy-Free Chocolate Pudding Recipe ✳
Sugar	Xylitol Sucanat – unrefined raw cane Erythritol
Crunchy Food	Apple and almonds Carrots dipped in guacamole Brown rice crackers Veggie Tortilla Wrap✳